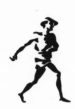

Coping with Your

by Natalie Golos
and Frances Golos Golbitz

Allergies

with Frances Spatz Leighton

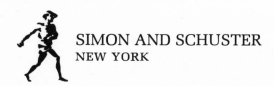

SIMON AND SCHUSTER
NEW YORK

Published by Simon and Schuster
A Division of Gulf & Western Corporation
Simon & Schuster Building
Rockefeller Center
1230 Avenue of the Americas
New York, New York 10020
SIMON AND SCHUSTER and colophon are trademarks
of Simon & Schuster
Designed by Irving Perkins
Manufactured in the United States of America
Printed and bound by Fairfield Graphics, Inc.
2 3 4 5 6 7 8 9 10 11

Library of Congress Cataloging in Publication Data

Golos, Natalie.
    Coping with your allergies.

    Bibliography: p.
    Includes index.
    1. Allergy. 2. Allergy-Prevention. I. Golbitz,
Frances Golos, joint author. II. Leighton, Frances
Spatz, joint author. III. Title.
RC584.G64   616.9'7   79-12366

ISBN 0-671-24078-1

To Mother Ida Siskin Golos
In Memoriam

CONTENTS

8   Contents

FOREWORD

THIS VOLUME is a significant improvement over previous guides for those with the problem of chemical susceptibility—commonly referred to as allergy—who wish to improve their lot. Miss Golos is to be commended in this endeavor; the book is more precise, detailed, and generally more applicable than previous efforts.

One of the most troublesome tasks of practicing clinical ecology is the tremendous time required in the education of patients. The word "education" is used advisedly because more than instruction and question answering is involved. Patients must be educated in both the philosophy and distinctive features of this type of medicine, as well as in the details of applying it. I will attempt to discuss the former, inasmuch as Miss Golos has done a good job with the latter.

Patients often inquire, shortly after they learn that they have a chemical susceptibility problem, "How and why did I suddenly get into this fix?" Although all the answers to this question are not available, some of them are. For instance, it is well known that the tendency to develop allergy or individual susceptibility is inherited, but that this exaggerated mode of response to one's environment may develop in anyone. The only point to emphasize here is that, from the standpoint of one's heredity, allergy develops more readily and seems to advance more rapidly in some people than in others.

The greatest single determinant in the development of this clinical problem concerns the environmental exposures themselves. These factors are best discussed under acute and chronic exposures—both of which are important.

Factors which apparently act to break or lower resistance, inducing acute reactions:

(1) Infection, particularly viral infections, will sometimes start the train of events leading to the chemical susceptibility problem. Measles, whooping cough, infectious mononucleosis, and shingles are examples of this factor.

(2) Hormone changes may act similarly. Women seem to be especially vulnerable immediately after pregnancy and at the change of life, although there tends to be some increased vulnerability premenstrually each month.

(3) A prolonged period of sleep deprivation or exhaustion may precipitate acute reactions.

(4) By far the most important cause of acute reactions and sustained susceptibility is massive chemical exposures. Although the first breakdown of resistance may follow a single massive chemical exposure, more commonly such exposures extend over a period of several days or weeks. A few examples will be described briefly.

A laboratory worker accidentally placed a bucket of liquid plastic on a hot stove. It exploded, filling the laboratory with toxic fumes. Out of several persons similarly exposed, this individual developed severe bronchospasm and asthma. Remaining unemployed and unemployable since, she has been forced to live in a rural area and has been unable to visit industrial areas.

A steelworker was forced to operate his crane in a steel mill while the ceiling and structural beams were being spray painted. He not only became acutely ill but, apparently as a result of this excessive exposure, he became so susceptible that he has been unemployable since that time.

An art student attended a pottery class in a large, poorly ventilated room in which on one side there was silk screening and oil painting, and on the other side a huge gas-fired kiln. After three weeks of such exposures, the onset of headaches, nausea, low-grade fever, and persistent asthma terminated that activity. A year later, she worked fourteen hours a day for a week with paints and paint removers while redecorating a large apartment containing a leaking gas range. Following those massive exposures, she remained bedridden for several months. Even though thirty years have elapsed since then, she remains extremely susceptible to a wide range of chemical environmental exposures despite living in a protected environment.

It is even more common to lose the ability to resist a wide variety of chemical environmental exposures if one is subjected to small amounts of low-grade chemical exposure over a sustained period of time.

One of the most common examples of such exposure, resulting in chronic manifestations, is that of housewives regularly exposed to the fumes of the unvented, gas-fired kitchen range. This kind of environmental exposure is rarely ever suspected, except if the health of such a person improves during a vacation only to have fatigue, headache, and/or arthritis recur within a few hours after returning home. Even then, the kitchen stove may not be identified as the cause.

There are many similar low-grade occupational exposures responsible for a slow, long-term buildup of individual susceptibility to environmental chemicals. This has been observed repeatedly in mechanics, printers, artists, painters, plastics workers, cooks, and others subjected to volatile hydrocarbons. Once individual susceptibility to a given facet of this chemical environmental problem develops, cross-reactions often spread to other related materials by the time the manifestations of illness prompt the victim to seek medical attention. Such developments often confuse observations of cause and effect.

It should be apparent to the reader that the medical approach involved here of demonstrating the environmental causes of chronic illness is not in the mainstream of current medical practice, which in general is directed more toward treating the effects of chronic ills than demonstrating and coping with their environmental causes. This book is of particular value to the person undergoing an ecologic evaluation and learning how to follow through with specific instructions.

The more one knows about the potentiality of this medical program, the better, and reading this book is a fine start. The book is good insurance to counteract the "Oh, that doesn't hurt, I can take it" attitude, so common among the great mass of undiagnosed chronically ill patients *before* they fall over the precipice.

Theron G. Randolph, M.D.

PREFACE

NO ONE loves living things more than we do. We are distressed if even a plant withers and dies. So our respect for life—all forms of living things—cannot be challenged.

Yet we are appalled at the fact that people interested enough to join organizations involved with environmental protection show enormous concern about our endangered animals with seldom a word for their endangered brothers and sisters—we of the human species. Surely human life is as dear and should be as valued as that of our animal friends.

"Clinical ecology is the study of an individual's reaction to his environment." That is the concise definition of the late Jonathan Forman, M.D., one of the founding fathers of the Society for Clinical Ecology.

To elaborate, man's environment includes the food he eats, the water he drinks, and the air he breathes in the places he lives, works, and plays.

Clinical ecology is a relatively new approach to medical practice, as yet largely untaught and unknown to most physicians. But an increasing number of physicians and other scientists are turning to clinical ecology, bringing to the subject a constant flow and interchange of ideas.

This book has been profoundly influenced by the clinical ecology movement. The present work is an outgrowth of two previous books, *Manual for Those Sensitive to Foods, Drugs and Chemicals* and *Management of Complex Allergies.*

Many of the clinical ecologists who made use of these two books for their patients with severe and complex allergies have concluded that countless conditions can be prevented, or at least greatly minimized, if people with minor sensitivities have prevention information readily available to them.

This book has been written to fulfill that need. It is a practical guide for the prevention and alleviation of allergies. It also teaches allergic individuals how to cope with their sensitivities and the overload of pollution in modern life. Finally, it shows those with minor complaints how to prevent such tendencies from developing into full-fledged allergies.

The materials gathered for this work have been compiled from the rich and varied experiences of many clinical ecologists and more significantly from countless individuals who have learned to cope with their problems.

However, the following must be singled out for special appreciation: Eloise Kailin, M.D., of Sequim, Washington, who initiated and provided guidance for the original work; Theron G. Randolph, M.D., of Chicago, William Rea, M.D., of Dallas, and Karl Humiston, M.D., of Sulphur Spring, Arkansas, who have contributed material, checked our work, and authenticated particular areas of medical expertise. Different chapters are the responsibility of different consultants, not all of whom use the same methods.

For their assistance in numerous ways, our special thanks to Jane Roller, Vera Rea, Audri Allred, Robert Ingram, Bonnie Rich Humiston, Iris Ingram, Beatrice Trum Hunter, Beth Kastonolis, Ruth Hagy Brod, and Dr. and Mrs. Carlton Fredericks.

Our thanks go as well to the members of the Society for Clinical Ecology, whose generous sharing of ideas has made it impossible to trace the original source of information. We extend our gratitude to the group as a whole.

In addition to the physicians mentioned in the text, we should like to give thanks to those who, though not directly quoted, have helped with interviews and answers to questions. Drs. Stevan Cordas, William Crook, Glen Green, Abram Hoffer, Harris Hosen, Vernon Jackson, Richard MacKarness, Vincent Mark, Joseph Miller, Douglas Sandberg, Ralph Smiley, Lendon H. Smith, Robert Vance, and James Whittington.

To Herman Golbitz, brother-in-law and husband, respectively, who was always there when we needed him, and who exhibited immeasurable patience, our thanks with love.

—Natalie Golos
—Frances Golbitz

A Note to the Mildly Allergic

If you are one of the millions of stuffy, drippy, or runny noses who treks periodically to the doctor to get your shot, you belong to this group. Perhaps you are one of those who tries to take care of oozing, itching, bloodshot eyes, muscle aches, or headaches by using over-the-counter medications that promise miraculous relief. You may belong to the class of the once-in-a-while rashes or hives.

As you read the book you will see that we are discussing prevention, management, and control of varying degrees of allergy. We are addressing not only your needs but also the needs of those who have no allergy problem but are health-oriented and therefore interested in prevention, those who are chronically ill and whose conditions remain undiagnosed because some doctors have not yet learned to relate these symptoms to allergy, and those who suffer numerous and severe reactions.

But our special message in this note is for you, all of you who know you have allergies, and either ignore them, or settle for shots and/or medicine.

First about the medicine: *Temporary relief hides symptoms.* Symptoms are warnings; pay heed to them. Medicine that relieves your nasal drip is no more a cure than the aspirin which temporarily relieves the pain and inflammation of arthritis. They do have one thing in common. Both are potentially dangerous with possible cumulative side effects. What is even worse, when that medicine ceases to give relief—aspirin, decongestant or whatever—and it eventually does, you may resort to something stronger and then something stronger again until you are really hooked.

Now, about shots; your doctor can help you only up to a point. The real help must come from you and your willingness to help yourself. That is the message of this book: what you can do by yourself for yourself to alleviate your reactions and to avoid more serious problems in the future.

PART I

A Guide for the Undiagnosed and the Mildly Allergic Person

CHAPTER 1

An Introduction to
Your Allergy Problems

HIDDEN ALLERGIES

ARE YOU one of those people who say, "I have no allergies—there is just one thing that bothers me"?

That phrase "just one" may be a clue. That one little thing that bothers you might trigger any one of a long list of conditions and illnesses that most people do not realize have any connection with allergies.

Environmental factors have been identified as causes of many forms of acute, chronic, and recurrent illness. Do you suffer from one or more of the following symptoms?
- Itching, flushing, burning or blistering of the skin?
- Fatigue, dizziness, numbness?
- Blurred vision, headaches, mental depression, poor concentration, behavior changes?
- Palpitations or skipped heartbeats?
- Excessive hunger, compulsive eating, or great thirst?
- Compulsive smoking?
- Stammering, stuttering, or hoarseness?
- Health problems such as arthritis, colitis, dermatitis, hypertension, migraine, obesity, alcoholism, epilepsy, colic, hives, urethral or bladder disorders, reading or writing disabilities, gastrointestinal disturbances or psoriasis?

This is only a partial listing of symptoms and health problems frequently related to allergy. This is not to imply that these conditions always are allergy related. But in many cases, they have been eliminated by removing the offending substances from the diet, from the water supply, or from the indoor or outdoor environment. Any tissue, organ or body system can be affected.

An incredible variety of *reversible* physical and mental disturbances can be caused by reactions to commonly encountered and generally unsuspected factors in the environment. Such symptoms and ailments may require the skillful services of a professional who practices clinical ecology.

As we pointed out in the Preface, clinical ecology is a new approach to medicine whereby man is examined in relation to his adaptation to his total environment. Because it is a new approach, foreign to most practitioners, and not yet taught in medical schools, it is frequently rejected by many dedicated doctors. Patients are often told, "There is nothing wrong with you . . . physically," implying that their ailment is psychosomatic. All too frequently, patients are referred to a psychiatrist in the mistaken belief that their symptoms suggest severe mental disturbance, when in reality the cause is hidden allergies.

One of the doctors who practices clinical ecology, Dr. Marshall Mandell, reported the case of a young man who was confined to a maximum security ward in a mental hospital and considered violent and uncontrollable. Dr. Mandell advised the attending psychiatrist to put the patient on a five-day fast, giving him only spring water.

A water fast, it should be explained, purges the system of all foods —including those that might be causing reactions. When foods are reintroduced one at a time, a clinical ecologist can determine whether or not the patient is allergic to it.

In this case, at the end of the five-day period the patient was "perfectly calm and pleasant." But when he was given eggs as the first food after the fast—a suspected offending food—he became so violent that it took five attendants to get him into a straitjacket. On the basis of this evidence, Dr. Mandell was able to determine that eggs were a contributing factor to the man's violent behavior.

Similarly, in cases of hyperactive children, or those with learning disabilities, blame is frequently placed upon guilt-ridden parents rather than on the true culprit: hidden allergies and sensitivities. The comment is often made, "There is nothing wrong with the child; perhaps it is the parent." Yet in many cases these conditions are symptomatic of an illness referred to as "chemical susceptibility" or "cerebral food allergy."

Physicians who are not yet educated to an understanding of the practices of clinical ecology frequently are baffled by various chronic illnesses, unaware that some patients should be tested in relation to environmental factors. If there is any persistent or recurrent condition still unresolved by the attending physician, it is recommended that a clinical ecologist be consulted.

Another indication of the need for such consultation is when the symptoms fall into recognizable patterns: Do the symptoms increase at a particular time of day? Or season of the year? Do they increase during a pollution alert? After eating? After shopping? While traveling? During work hours? At school? Such recurring symptoms should be viewed as clues to possible environmental causes.

Sometimes people are too busy to pay attention to what they consider minor problems. Or they may have been so brainwashed about psychosomatic illness that they dismiss minor isolated discomfort, having been taught that it is a sign of courage and strength of character to "grin and bear it." This book, it is hoped, will convince the reader that it is not courageous but rather foolhardy to ignore pain and discomfort.

In addition to clinical ecologists, government officials are currently expressing concern over the impact of environmental factors on health. Douglas M. Costle, in assuming his role as administrator of the Environmental Protection Agency (EPA), stated that he considered the implementation of the Toxic Substances Control Act as "one of the most difficult challenges and important priorities facing EPA," and ordered an investigation of fifteen substances considered possible risks to public health.

"We have neglected the subtle, but lethal, effects of chemicals for decades," Costle went on to say. "Now we must extend the frontiers of public knowledge to find out what these risks really are and find ways to control them. . . . Our society must take any needed precautions to prevent the occurrence of silent epidemics."

If you have any skepticism about the relation of environmental factors to a wide range of health problems, check it out yourself. The next time an extended pollution period is announced, ask relatives, friends, fellow workers, and especially persons employed by or living in the vicinity of industrial plants, about the following:

Is there any increase in absenteeism (for example, among mechanics and road construction workers)?

Is there increased fatigue and irritability (especially in heavy traffic)?

Is there any increase in minor complaints such as eye, ear, nose, or throat irritation? Chest pressure? Stomach disorders or nausea? Dizziness? Headaches? Other irritations?

Once, after a ten-day period labeled as "hazardous air," we found the following had occurred: A local hospital had an increased number of emergency admissions, including automobile accidents, accidents in the home, and illnesses not necessarily related to lung and heart disease (which are known to be aggravated by air pollution). A local social service office and the police department reported increases in cases of child abuse, wife beating, and other social crimes. A local school reported increased disciplinary problems. These results were not surprising. The toxins in the air have been demonstrated time and again to cause many problems of this kind.

As an illustration of mental confusion caused by air pollution there is the classic example of Florence, a woman who is extremely well organized, and who thinks and writes clearly and precisely. She is also an excellent athlete, very well coordinated. During a pollution alert, however, she becomes disorganized, fumbles for words, writes like a grade school student, bumps into everything, and in general has such poor coordination that her golf and tennis games appear to be those of a beginner.

Florence's experience illustrates the correlation between the mind and the body, between mental and physical health.

That also brings to mind a woman who thought she was suffering from arthritis. Then she went to India, where she escaped the smoke and chemical pollution of the big cities in the United States—particularly New York, where she spent most of her time—and her arthritis disappeared. When she returned home, her arthritis recurred.

During any extended period of hazardous air, note what minor complaints you have experienced, or illnesses and irritations that formerly you never associated with air pollution.

A minor chronic discomfort might be a warning which if unheeded can develop into a serious situation. Jeanne had minor backaches that were at first uncomfortable enough to be a constant annoyance but not serious enough to cause alarm. She attributed the pains to an injury sustained during a high school basketball game. Her backaches grew worse, but she still thought that nothing could be done about them because of that old injury. However, when she was tested for a totally different complaint, her doctor discovered that she was allergic to yeast. The backaches stopped when Jeanne discontinued eating foods containing yeast. Fortunately, she did not have to give up breadstuffs altogether; she simply substituted unleavened breads like matzos and various crackers, and learned to bake others without yeast.

Almost anything with which a person comes in contact can become an excitant, the thing that causes a reaction. Mary was afflicted with itching around the eyes. The problem was so annoying that she went to an allergist, one who was not familiar with clinical ecology. After a routine battery of tests everything proved negative, indicating no allergies.

Mary knew that something was bothering her, but the pattern was so erratic that she could not detect the excitant. The discomfort was constant, but there were periods when the itching was more severe than usual. Each day the period of severity varied in frequency and duration, but seemed at its worst in the morning. The allergist referred Mary to an opthalmologist, who labeled the problem "eye strain." The medication that he prescribed did not ease the itching but instead created side effects. (It was later learned that the medication contained phenol, a preservative to which she was sensitive.)

Other symptoms began to appear. Mary developed pain in the eyes, swollen lids, inability to focus, and weeping eyes. Some time later she discovered that her condition was caused by fumes from newsprint. Now, as long as she doesn't handle the newspaper, her eyes remain normal.

At this point it is important to emphasize once again that the symptoms discussed in this chapter are not *always* caused by foods, drugs, inhalants, or other environmental factors. Not all illnesses are allergy related. But allergy is an area likely to be overlooked, and one that needs to be explored.*

There are countless unfortunate people walking around in misery and pain because of illnesses that would disappear or be greatly alleviated if the people knew what to eliminate from their diets or their environment. When clinical ecology becomes better known and suitable treatment available to more people, life will be much more comfortable and worth living for many whose illnesses remain a mystery.

Some years ago, a fifth-grade child named Lisa, in apparent good health, complained of discomfort when getting in and out of her desk seat. Since this occurred only during art class, the teacher, knowing the child disliked that particular subject, assumed her condition to be psychosomatic.

The teacher even teased the little girl, referring to her as "my little old lady with the rheumatiz." Unfortunately, those pains which were being ignored were warning signals. Today, as an adult, Lisa knows what caused the pain. She has crippling pain whenever she is exposed to paint.

Another case in point involves a woman, Deborah, who had been sickly all her life—except when she took a trip to Italy. It wasn't until she returned, grew worse, and was put into a hospital in Texas that she discovered the reason for the magic of Italy. While a patient, it was learned that among other things Deborah reacted to the paints, treated wall board and other toxic substances in the walls. In Italy, the rooms where she stayed had walls made of marble, an inert material.

As mentioned previously, clinical ecology is a pioneer field of med-

* The interested physician who wishes to investigate this field in detail is referred to *Clinical Ecology*, the textbook on this subject, edited by Dr. Lawrence Dickey,[1] and *Human Ecology and Susceptibility to the Chemical Environment*, by Dr. T. G. Randolph,[2] the original pioneer in this field and the first to recognize chemical susceptibility as a prime cause of many chronic debilitating diseases.

icine. But there is evidence that this approach has worked in thousands upon thousands of cases where patients had previously been told there was no hope.

Since there are case histories of hundreds of persons suffering from arthritis who found relief through clinical ecology, why not test arthritics for environmental causes before plying them with medication such as aspirin which could aggravate the condition?

Why shouldn't it be routine procedure to test alcoholics for grain allergies, when it is known that many alcoholics are addicted to a particular grain and have been helped by learning to avoid it?

Why shouldn't it be routine practice to test schizophrenics for environmental factors, when there are case histories showing the relation of adverse environmental conditions to symptoms of schizophrenia?

Some of the practices discussed in the section of this book on nontoxic living may at first glance seem far-fetched. Some may sound reasonable only to a person who knows how difficult it is to buy a mattress without materials in it that will make him ill. And they will sound reasonable enough to the mother who searched for some kind of a contraption like the reading box mentioned in Chapter 19, "Tips for the Beginner," so that her daughter would be able to do her schoolwork.

Allergy sufferers have told us many times that they never appreciated modern conveniences until they suddenly found they had to do without them. For example, when one woman became ill, she had to resort to using several pans of costly spring water to wash her vegetables. After years of moving from place to place in search of a clean environment, she built a house at great expense to provide nontoxic living. The convenience she enjoyed most in her new home was the filter on her faucet (see Chapter 23). It was so good to be able to wash her vegetables under running water again—something most people take for granted.

For those of you who are using this book for prevention rather than management of allergies, it will at least alert you to the kinds of things you should be looking for in order to clear up the pollution in your home.

What worries us a great deal is the irresponsibility of governmental control agencies concerned with pesticides and other chemical agents who claim that the public is effectively protected. The informed person knows this cannot be true, but the general public remains blissfully unaware unless personally afflicted.

As we kill off insects with ever greater amounts of pesticides, we may also be killing ourselves. There is even a name for it: ecolocide.

That's what Frances Silver, a noted ecologic consulting engineer, calls the method of destroying man by slowly altering the environment.

As for how serious the problem of pesticides is, Dr. Theron Randolph, the father of clinical ecology, says:

"The next worst pollutant besides gas utilities are pesticide residues. Houses which have been exterminated regularly should be put up for sale, as one will never get over it.

"You cannot be completely certain that you have ever eliminated the most pernicious pesticides from an insecticide-treated house. With the new Toxic Substances Control Act, we may be in a much stronger position to nail down these exposures which we thought were innocuous. We may be in a position to bring to bear some of our views.

"The EPA is very much interested in patients reporting to them on their experiences."

This book contains many sources for buying nontoxic products, and lists brand names as well. It is a sad commentary on the state of affairs that people have had to combine their efforts for over ten years to find the sources mentioned in this book, sources of nontoxic materials and products that are needed for everyday use. It is often necessary to write to some distant place, or even order them from foreign countries.

Although we have tried hard to include only those products that have proven helpful to many sensitive people, each person must test the product for himself. This must be done for two reasons: first, *no product is safe for everyone;* second, products safe at the time this goes to press may become contaminated tomorrow because the manufacturer has decided to "improve" the product. We have learned to look with suspicion on any product that is marked "new" or "improved."

The layman interested in more information on environmental problems can contact the Human Ecology Action League (HEAL), a national nonprofit organization whose primary aim is to educate its members, the medical community, and the public at large by making available information about illness caused by the environment.

The organization was originally formed at the request of hundreds of patients who had suffered needlessly for years before discovering a clinical ecologist who recognized the causes of their illnesses. These patients, wanting to help others avoid their own misfortunes, have urged the formation of a central data collection pool. The address is: HEAL, 505 North Lakeshore Drive, Suite 6506, Chicago, Illinois 60611.

Numbered among the HEAL membership from the field of medicine are general practitioners, allergists, internists, pediatricians, otolaryngologists, opthalmologists, surgeons, and psychiatrists (many of whom are practitioners in the field of clinical ecology). For help in locating a local physician who is especially interested in the environmental factors in human illness, contact Dr. Del Stigler, Secretary of the Society for Clinical Ecology, 2005 Franklin, Suite 490, Denver, Colorado 80205.

CHAPTER 2

Allergy, Sensitivity, Addiction—What's It All About?

STOP. BEFORE you go any further, let's clear up an important point. When you take this book to show your doctor, and we hope all of you do, he may very likely tell you that we don't know what we're talking about—that what we are discussing are not allergies.

Well, technically he's right. But technically, we're right too.

Historically, the word "allergy" came from two Greek words, *állos* meaning "altered" or "other," and *érgon* meaning "work" or "action." It was Dr. Clement Von Perquet, an Austrian pediatrician, who came up with the word "allergy." Originally, an allergic person was considered to be one who had a reaction to something which does not affect other people.

Over the years, the diagnosis and treatment of allergy have become more specialized. To understand the nature of allergies, you must become acquainted with the words "antibody" and "antigen." Antibodies are a protein produced by the human body to match a particular foreign substance called an antigen. Once the antibody is formed and the antigen is reintroduced to the human body, the combination can cause harm to one or more tissues of the body.

The scratch test is widely used in classical allergy to ascertain which antigens cause harm. Dr. Hobart Feldman, of North Miami Beach, Florida, a past president of the Society for Clinical Ecology, formerly used the scratch testing in his allergy practice, but he found it was not accurate enough for definitive diagnosis and treatment. It is worthless for the migraine equivalent resulting from foods, and most drugs and chemicals.

The migraine equivalent is a form of cerebral allergy in which blood vessels in the brain are the target. Fluid escaping from blood vessels and lymph glands results in edema: the fluids pile up in the tissues, swelling the brain in the same way that ankles swell after an injury or your nose swells during hay fever season.

These symptoms are similar because they indicate an intolerance to something. An allergy is an intolerance; a chemical sensitivity is also an intolerance. That is why we use the words "allergy" and "sensitivity" interchangeably.

With the proliferation of synthetic chemicals in air, water, food—in our total environment—the clinical ecologists have returned to the broader meaning of allergy. Thus, if we wanted to be technical with today's interpretation, instead of using the word "allergy" it would be more accurate to describe these conditions, these reactions, as *sensitivities, susceptibilities,* and *intolerances.*

We intend to use those terms interchangeably. When we speak of allergies we shall be using the historic definition—a reaction to something that does not necessarily affect other people.

Excuse us for being personal, but this is the only way we can express our reason for making the decision to use "allergy" in the broadest sense. Someone very close to us happens to be one individual who fits into both classifications: she suffers from the classical allergic reactions which involve antibodies, as well as the type which today should technically be called chemical susceptibilities and food sensitivities.

She is just as sick either way, and she couldn't care less what it is called. She is just grateful to the allergists who, because they included clinical ecology in their practice, have been able to help her.

The problem with chemical susceptibilities and food sensitivities is that you need to be a detective to discover them. In order to understand the reason for this, you have to know the meaning of "masked sensitivity and addiction."

The best way to explain "masked sensitivity" is to take a familiar example. Almost everyone who has ever smoked a cigarette can recall that with his first cigarette he had some sort of reaction—he coughed, he became a little dizzy, or he felt queasy. After a few cigarettes he no longer had a problem. Or at least he thought he no longer had a problem. In reality, the symptoms were masking themselves.

This can be explained in the same way with foods. Infants frequently react to their foods with colic, irritability, or skin rash. After a time, the symptoms seem to disappear just as the doctor had predicted: "The child will outgrow it." Regrettably, that's not always true. Instead of outgrowing it, the child may be showing signs of masked sensitivity.

This unfortunately leads to addiction. To understand food addiction, think of drug addiction. It's the same process. You become accustomed to a certain food, you develop a need for the food, you create a craving for the food.

To cite an example: a woman who was being tested for food sensitivities told the doctor that he didn't have to test her for eggs because she ate them all the time. She reported that whenever she had a migraine, she ate eggs and soon felt some relief.

The fact is, the eggs were a fix, just as heroin is a fix to a heroin addict. It relieved the symptoms, but only temporarily. And within a short time, she would begin to crave the eggs again.

Hers was a typical food addiction. The longer it continues, the more addicted you can become. And the more addicted you become, the more muddy your medical picture becomes. The symptoms begin to mount up.

Because eggs are in other foods, the person addicted to eggs finds that he craves other things as well. One example is pastries. So he begins eating more and more pastries, which usually are made with wheat. And then he begins to crave bread, and so on and on until he has developed multiple food allergies—addiction—with such a variety of symptoms that he goes from specialist to specialist, creating the impression that he is a hypochondriac.

In the case of the woman with the egg addiction, it was not difficult for the clinical ecologist to pinpoint the troublemaker. This is true also with the individual who says, "In the morning I'm as mean as a bull until I have my cup of coffee." This almost certainly indicates a coffee addiction. (So does the situation with the individual who reports, "My nerves are so shattered, I must have a cigarette.") Unfortunately, when there is a series of masked sensitivities, the causes of the symptoms are not so obvious, and it may take the clinical ecologist longer to determine what is giving his patient the fix.

Dr. William Rea, noted cardiovascular surgeon of Dallas, Texas, uses the term "environmentally triggered disease" to explain masked allergies. He compares the body's response to a barrel being filled with water. If you put in one drop more than the barrel will hold, it will spill over. Stress in the body is absorbed in the same way. If you subject the body to more stress than it can handle, it will spill over and illness results.

This is not to say that all stress is harmful. We need stress. Lack of stress can be harmful, and we would sit around like vegetables without it. It's all a matter of balance.

Food is a stress because it starts the digestive tract reacting. Air is a stress because it activates the lungs and heart. Under normal circumstances, they are healthy stresses. However, when the body is exposed to abnormal stresses which act like poison to the system, then they are unhealthy stresses.

When you continue to add food poisons and air pollutants to the normal stresses of life, the time comes when you have one stress too many and the body is taxed beyond its ability to adapt. Suddenly you have an environmentally triggered disease which erupts into chronic illness such as constant headaches, depression, arthritis, vascular problems, or skin rashes. Something sort of explodes, and the slight sensitivity to cigarette smoke or perfume or paint or certain foods causes an overflow like the barrel of water spilling over. You finally find yourself unable to tolerate the slightest exposure to almost any chemical and, believe it or not, to any food.

Can you imagine not being able to tolerate any food you eat? Such a person is called a "universal food reactor." Fortunately, even universal food reactors can be restored to good health in the skillful hands of a clinical ecologist.

What sets the clinical ecologist apart from most other physicians is that the former takes into account the fact that the triggering stress is biological rather than psychological in nature.

Clinical ecologists are linking chemical susceptibilities to all kinds of illnesses for which, at the present time, traditional medicine has no satisfactory treatment. Chronic illnesses such as schizophrenia, manic depression, urinary disorder, or arthritis can sometimes be reversed merely by removing the excitants—the causal agents—and then adding them back under controlled conditions.

In a report to the Society for Clinical Ecology in November, 1975, Dr. F. Murray Carroll of Chadbourn, North Carolina, who has studied more than a hundred patients with different kinds of arthritis, told of a thirty-one-year-old woman who was bedridden with arthritic pain so severe it could not be controlled by the recognized salicylate and steroid treatment. Dr. Carroll found the woman to be sensitive to ten foods. After eliminating these foods from her diet, she had only three flare-ups during the sixteen months she was being studied. Each time she had a flare-up, it was because she had eaten a food to which she was sensitive.

Dr. Carroll reported that of his hundred cases, about half became almost symptom-free after the offending foods were removed from the diet and another 30 percent were "substantially" improved.

Dr. Carroll admitted that he was having tough-sledding trying to convince his colleagues in the local hospital that there could be a connection between allergies and arthritis. A job needs to be done on educating doctors, and more will be said about that later.

We wonder how long it will take the Arthritis Foundation to support research in this area. This is not a new concept, and research support for it is long past due.

In 1934, Dr. Michael Zeller was the first to publish a paper in a medical journal reporting the effect of foods on arthritis. Later, Dr.

Randolph associated chemicals and arthritis. For many years, Dr. Randolph has been successfully treating many arthritic patients—even those with rheumatoid arthritis—through environmental control and the rotary diversified diet (see Chapter 8).

Children can be as vulnerable as adults. Often, when a child shows irritability for no apparent reason, a food is at the bottom of it.

Most of the time Billy was gentle as a lamb and did not make a fuss about anything. But suddenly, a perverse streak seemed to surface and he would be a complete brat. Not only that, but when he was in his bratty periods, he would refuse to do anything that taxed his mind, such as working a puzzle or doing homework. When peaches were tested positive—meaning he was allergic to them—and were removed from the diet, his behavior improved.

Some cases of child abuse have been recognized as the result of both child and parent reacting to their allergies at the same time. One such mother said in tears that her greatest joy is that now she recognizes when her child is reacting to excitants and she can cope with him in spite of her own allergies. She wishes his teacher could understand when his naughty behavior is triggered by the toxins in the classroom.

Some children exhibit recognizable allergic symptoms such as sneezing, runny nose, and respiratory problems. Others have symptoms such as vomiting, diarrhea, and bed wetting, which are not so easily diagnosed. And, like adults, children can have an addiction to certain foods.

Chuck was a classic case of food addiction. He would go to a neighborhood store and buy several kinds of chocolate cookies and chocolate candy and gobble them all down in the space of an hour. He would be sick the next day, but as soon as he had money he would do the same thing. Some days Chuck would come home from school and become hysterical, screaming for something to eat.

It was found that Chuck's craving for chocolate was an addiction. When he couldn't have chocolate, he suffered withdrawal symptoms, much in the manner of a drug addict withdrawing from drugs.

Certain people suffer from multiple sensitivities, and when such reports appear in a newspaper or magazine, we find that the reporter has assumed that this is unique. Many if not most readers believe it to be so. Unfortunately, this is not an unusual circumstance. It is possible for an individual to be so allergic to pollens, synthetics, automobile exhaust, cigarette smoke, as well as other pollutants in the air that he must find a place to escape to. Some people have found a trip to the seashore beneficial because there the breezes off the water tend to cleanse the air and make breathing more tolerable.

This is only a temporary form of relief. Some persons have had to leave school, change jobs, retire or resign from a job, and some have found it necessary to move to a healthier environment to obtain permanent relief. It is impossible to estimate how many people suffer allergies in this way. The real question is how many suffer multiple allergies but don't know it because their susceptibilities are masked and have remained undiagnosed.

When the scratch test is not valid, what test can be used? The best method is called comprehensive environmental control—avoidance followed by challenge—which is most effectively accomplished in a hospital ecologic unit which has been cleared of toxic substances.

During a fast allowing only pure spring water, the body is virtually purged of all toxins. After this "avoidance," the patient is given a meal consisting of one food, organically grown and unseasoned except for salt. This is called "challenge," and must be done when the patient's system has been freed of the effect of masking.

The validity of environmental control testing can be illustrated by relating the case of a woman whose major admitting complaint was diarrhea. After a fast, all her symptoms, including the diarrhea, had cleared. For her first food after the fast, she was given salmon. Before she had finished eating, the diarrhea returned.

We are relating this not because it's a unique case, but to show the reliability of this cause-and-effect type of testing. Nothing else had changed in her environment, and the only food in her system, the only new thing introduced to her, was the salmon.

An interesting sidelight to this test was reported by the patient. As she was eating the salmon, her nose became so stuffed she found it difficult to breathe, to speak, or even to continue eating; she had to breathe through her mouth. To this day, she's quite amused and still amazed as she recalls what happened to her. She says, "As the contents gushed from my system, my nose simultaneously miraculously cleared."

There are other challenge procedures, such as the provocative sublingual test, in which an extract of the substance being tested is placed under the tongue. The principle here is the same as in the case of nitroglycerine for angina. The substance is absorbed more quickly into the system because it is placed under the tongue.

A film of such a food test administered in a physician's office showed fascinating results. Five minutes after a particular food extract was placed under the patient's tongue, she went into a catatonic state, unable to move a muscle or communicate. When this doctor stretched her arm up, it remained suspended in midair. When she was given a relieving dose treatment, a regulated quantity of the offending extract, she returned to her normal state.

Dr. Doris Rapp, a pediatric allergist of Buffalo, New York, an author of books about children's allergies, told us of double-blind studies she has made to validate these tests in which neither the patient nor the physician knows what, if anything, is being tested.[1] Sometimes a placebo is used—with no test material, only a saline solution. Mothers seeing their children provoked into hyperactive states right in front of their own eyes could correctly identify the testing extract as opposed to the placebo.

In another film, Dr. Clifton Brooks, a clinical ecologist of Tustin, California, is shown testing an infant for corn. He was using the Rinkel test, which is done with a needle intradermally (between the layers of the skin). The child, lying quietly in her mother's arms, began crying and showing signs of pain and discomfort. You could say, of course, the needle made him cry. If that were true, why did the needle containing the relieving dose of corn quiet the child?

Corn extract is given to the patient, provoking symptoms. Some doctors say that the correct dose of the same corn extract can sometimes help relieve symptoms, if the correct dose can be determined. An analogy can be drawn here to other medical procedures. Dust extract is used to desensitize a dust-sensitive patient. Vaccines are used to immunize against specific diseases.

There are other forms of testing. Chapter 8, "The Rotary Diversified Diet," teaches you to test foods, and Chapter 17, "How to Detect the Problem," explains how to test at home for chemicals.

Almost anything you can name can affect you. Perhaps the biggest shocker is that doctors have been finding that many patients are allergic to different kinds of water. Some patients have had to test eight or nine different kinds of water before they could find one they could tolerate.

People who have eaten a hearty meal and are soon hungry again show symptoms of a food sensitivity. The meal probably contained a food that caused symptoms similar to hunger pangs.

To illustrate food sensitivity, we'll use the story of Caroline, who always had hunger pangs in the middle of the night. She would go downstairs and raid the refrigerator. During the day she could never satisfy her hunger. When she grew older and became a severely sensitive individual, she discovered she was allergic to most of the foods she was eating. Since she has been tested, however, she can eat three meals a day and feel satisfied if she stays on her rotary diet.

If she had known that hunger can be a symptom, Caroline could have begun to practice the rotary diversified diet at the point when extreme hunger was her only symptom and perhaps avoided the severe allergies she developed.

If people become tired and fall asleep after meals, it is highly likely that some food they have just eaten—food to which they are allergic—has caused their fatigue and drowsiness.

Some people suffer from strong body odor and drench themselves with deodorants. The odor may be caused by certain foods or the contaminants in the food. One patient commented, "The only time I feel the need for a deodorant is when I have broken my diet by eating nonorganic foods."

Of course, there are certain foods, like onions or garlic, which have a strong odor and will give a person bad breath or body odor for a certain length of time. When you eat onions, garlic, or lamb, which happen to be foods that do cause an odor, make sure you eat a lot of parsley or comfrey, which are natural deodorants.

As for body odor, baking soda is such a good natural deodorant that it can be used as a body deodorant as well as a room deodorant. However, some people may find that it causes an irritation. If you break out in a rash, it may be because of the coarse texture of the baking soda. To correct this, put a cup of starch—cornstarch, arrowroot, tapioca, etc.—into the blender with a cup of baking soda and blend into a fine substance. You should then be able to use it without a problem.

Most people don't realize that children can be just as allergic to cigarette smoke as adults are. And children who are allergic to cigarette smoke can also be allergic to other pollutants in the air.

Robert was such a child. He went through the first and second grades and always did well in school, but he had respiratory trouble. In the fourth grade, when the school put in a new air conditioning system, he started getting so sick that he missed about two months out of the school year. In the sixth grade, Robert was sick most of the time.

In desperation, Robert's mother studied the layout of the school to see what was wrong. She discovered that the door to the incinerator was kept open much of the time and the smoke was reaching Robert's classroom. Unfortunately, the school also had installed a faulty cleaning system which scattered the dust instead of suctioning it. When the children came to school in the morning, dust covered everything.

As a final blow to his respiratory system, all Robert's teachers smoked, and the smoke bothered him very much. In the sixth grade, what had been considered moderately severe bronchitis became full-blown asthma. Robert had periods of dry coughing, wheezing, a tight feeling in the chest, and inability to breathe. His mother took him out of school, and he finished the year under the guidance of a visiting teacher.

Fortunately, the next year his mother was able to find a private school that was fairly uncontaminated. He did very well again in his classes, as long as he stayed out of the lunchroom. Robert's mother found that a gas stove adjoining the lunchroom through an archway was the culprit.

By rearranging his schedule, Robert was able to take all his courses in the morning, come home for lunch, and spend the rest of the day at home studying. He finished that year on the honor roll.

CHAPTER 3

The Prevention of Allergies

WE USED to hate those "world-coming-to-an-end people." We scoffed at Rachel Carson and her "silent spring."

What should we do, run and hide from life? Stop living? Stop eating?

For the past few years we've been eating those words letter by letter.

Today's simple reaction to toxic substances may be tomorrow's complex problem. A past president of the Society for Clinical Ecology, Dr. Eloise Kailin, explains it as follows: "It is wise to take heed of today's slight reaction to cosmetics, detergents, gasoline fumes, nylon, paint, or other toxic matter, for this is often the first indication of more serious trouble to come."

At the outset that presents a problem: unless people have been trained to do so, they are frequently not able to associate their reactions with the substance causing the upset.

If nylon or other synthetics make a person itch or break out, he is lucky in one respect; he is reacting to an *obvious* contact irritant. Unfortunately, most people do not know that the fumes of synthetics—detectable or not—are toxic and could be causing a reaction such as itching eyes, runny nose, or headache.

All of these toxic substances are foreign to the human body. When the body reaches its saturation level, it can no longer tolerate even minute exposure to that particular chemical.[1] Since ours is a chemically pregnant environment, the body, weakened by one chemical, builds up intolerances to multiple chemicals.

That is our second dilemma. Even chemical companies and other big industries which are the greatest contributors to pollution agree that the chemicals being introduced into our environment are poisonous and become dangerous at certain levels. The controversy rages over what level is dangerous. Is anyone qualified to make that determination?

When an "expert" recognizes the danger of a particular poison in a product but maintains that the level of toxicity is "safe," his position can be challenged by the use of one word, "overloading," a term used by clinical ecologists. "Overloading" can best be explained by citing an example of a patient who could tolerate milk until the ragweed season, at which time one glass of milk would clobber him. The patient, suffering from hay fever, had a mild allergy to milk. By itself, milk didn't bother him. It was the combination of excitants, one ingested and one inhaled, that made him ill.[2]

That's the point that is neglected in the arguments of experts who label poison at a "safe" level. The expert may be isolated in the laboratory with one toxic product; the public is not. The public is exposed to thousands of these products. The tragedy is that the overloading is so rampant that no one person has control over the amount of his exposure. Even the most careful individual is exposed to pollution in the air he breathes, the water he drinks, the food he eats.

That is why we need to take preventive measures. Until the public is awakened and clamors for change, the only recourse an individual has is to learn how to minimize his exposure. The following experiences of chemically susceptible patients illustrate the need for using preventive measures. To demonstrate why even minor symptoms should not be ignored, we will relate the story of a young woman whom we shall call Grace.

Grace learned in 1958 that she had allergies, but her physician told her they were so minor there was no need for her to see an allergist. Two years later she experienced a mild reaction to a certain deodorant, which caused swelling, and a few reactions to other things, but she ignored the symptoms for fear of being called a hypochondriac. By 1966 she was so ill she was unable to tolerate a normal diet and needed to move six times in her search for an environment she could tolerate.

It took just eight years for her condition to develop from a simple reaction to a semi-invalid state of complex allergies and severe chemical sensitivities.

"If I knew then what I know now," Grace complained, "maybe I could have predicted my worsening condition, and probably could have prevented at least the severity of the problem.

"The physicians who tried to help me were puzzled by the symptoms I could no longer ignore. An ophthalmologist told me that my blurred vision was probably caused by eye strain. My general practitioner said my chronic fatigue was caused by overwork. An internist-allergist said my problem could be a spastic colon. Finally, when I went to another allergist, I was given dust shots that contained preservatives. While I am still allergic to dust, one of my worst offenders is preservatives, especially the phenol in the dust extract.

"There can be no question that my sensitivity advanced from a mild to a severe degree because of what clinical ecologists call 'an overloading of the offenders.' "

To cite a few examples of overloading in Grace's case, let's examine her habits:

Food: Grace indulged her insatiable hunger for beef, potatoes, bread, and sweets. When her allergic condition was diagnosed, it was discovered that her worst food offenders were beef, potatoes, wheat, and sugar.

Chemicals: She was in the habit of wrapping everything in plastic, all her foods, everything in her closets and drawers: shoes, gloves, hats, sweaters, coats. She introduced other chemicals into her bedroom by installing bookshelves to hold books, magazines, ditto paper, carbon paper, felt-tip markers, and other toxic office supplies. It was later discovered that her most severe chemical reactions were induced by ink and plastics.

"In retrospect," Grace says, "while I am very grateful that my state of health improves weekly, regrets must intrude. If I had known in advance, I could probably have avoided the excitants which eventually overloaded my system and made me so ill."

So often people cannot really identify what is bothering them. A woman business executive we know of attended many banquets and dinners. She assumed she was allergic to flowers because she always sat on the dais and was exposed to them, and it was after these events that she felt ill. She has since discovered that she is allergic to nothing natural and that flowers do not bother her. It was the insecticide sprayed on the flowers that caused her problems.

Some people react to certain foods with indigestion or headaches, others break out in hives. One woman had suffered from hives for many years until she entered an ecologic unit in a hospital to find out where the trouble lay. She seemed not to be allergic to any foods until she was tested for pork, right after which she blossomed out in the most awful and painful case of hives.

She had liked pork and eaten quite a bit of it, but once she knew that this was a food addiction and was bad for her, she stayed away from it and was soon able to report that for the first time in over fifteen years she had clear skin and no longer had to use salves or medications.

Some time later she tried pork again, thinking that a little would not hurt. But again she had the ugly rash and pain from hives, and realized that she was through with pork forever.

Corn allergy is one of the most common food allergies. Jane, a doctor's wife, would sometimes be so irritable that she could hardly function and her children were not permitted to have friends visit. "Having them around just drove me up the wall," she said. "I could never understand why.

"Then when I started being tested for food allergies, one of the first tests was for corn. Immediately after I was injected with the corn preparation, I got all my symptoms again. I was nervous and irritable. My joints hurt, my head ached, and I just had this horrible feeling of agitation, like my body inside, outside, every place, was just vibrating. I was afraid if they didn't give me something very soon, they would have to scrape me off the ceiling.

"I felt so bad I wanted to scream. I never have been hit like that before. The doctor started giving me food shots, and I eliminated corn from my diet."

But once a person has developed a strong allergic reaction to a food, it isn't necessary to swallow it in order to get a reaction from it, as Jane discovered in her problem with corn allergy:

"I went to a movie weeks after I no longer ate corn products and I came out of the movie hurting all over just as I used to do when I ate corn. And then I realized I had been in there smelling popcorn for several hours—I was getting the same symptoms from smelling it as eating it."

Allergies produce different symptoms in different people. With milk, for example, some people get severe headaches. In others, it causes a sore throat or blocked ears. Some people become sleepy or irritable. Some suffer abdominal pain. Some become very depressed and have crying spells. Milk can cause the stomach cramps commonly referred to in infants as colic. Hives, too, have been traced to a milk allergy.

It is not unusual for food intolerance to be closely related to the buildup of chemical sensitivity. This was true for Marie, a botanist who was active and healthy until shortly after she began working for the Forest Service. The first thing that happened, she recalls, is that when she went into work she was bothered by the strong odor of paradichlorobenzine. She began having trouble with her eyes and severe pains in her joints. Then she got diarrhea, and as she put it, "crazy things started happening to me that had never happened before." The reaction became so bad that she couldn't read. She began having dizzy spells.

Other people noticed the awful smell of the paradichlorobenzine. "How can you stand it?" they would ask. It suddenly occurred to her that she couldn't even smell it anymore.

That is an important point. If you smell something and it bothers you and then it stops bothering you, it's too late for preventive measures because the damage has been done. The key to prevention is as soon as you smell a strong odor that bothers you, you must get rid of it immediately.

In this case, Marie did not act soon enough and the case became more complicated. At a later date a shipment of dried plants arrived from a different part of the country. They had been powdered with an insecticide that apparently affected her, because her fingertips became dry, her hands became swollen and stiff with pink splotches, and gradually she developed a severe arthritic condition.

She went to an arthritis specialist, who labeled it acute arthritis and treated her with gold shots. She kept getting stiffer and stiffer, and every joint in her body hurt. After a year and a half of these treatments, Marie realized that she was not getting any better; if anything, she was getting worse. It finally reached a point where she couldn't work, and she applied for disability pay.

Implying that it must be in her mind, a doctor working for the government tested her thoroughly and said he couldn't find anything wrong with her, and that there was no reason for her to receive disability pay. She had no alternative but to retire from her job. The government was willing to allow her to retire and receive 60 percent of her salary on disability if it were noted officially that there was a mental involvement. She refused: "I didn't do it because I didn't want to be labeled mentally disturbed."

Even today, Marie suffers from severe chest pains when confronted by certain chemicals. Yet in a clear environment she can go mountain climbing without any problem. She is not even out of breath while people younger than she are panting, trying to keep up with her. On her own street, however, she often cannot walk two blocks from her home to a mailbox because of her chest pains from traffic air pollution.

Marie's sensitivity to chemicals spilled over into an intolerance to foods. She has discovered that foods ordinarily tolerated in pure air become troublesome in polluted areas. For people like Marie, minimal intolerance becomes maximum intolerance under these conditions. Once they move to a clear environment, such people frequently find they are no longer allergic to certain foods.

This situation further strengthens the case against overloading—and the need for prevention.

Prevention should begin with children. Adults don't realize how frequently children are affected by hidden allergies. How often does a psychologist or psychiatrist delve into the ecologic reasons that an older child wets his bed? Clinical ecologists have discovered that, for example, bed wetting can be caused by allergies. One doctor we know learned this cause and effect with his own daughter. Sandra was still wetting the bed at the age of six, even though the doctor and his wife were careful to take her to the bathroom before putting her to bed and to restrict her liquid intake in the evening.

After careful observation, the parents realized that any day Sandra ate oranges or grapes, she was sure to wet the bed. They tested the theory and came to the conclusion that a sensitivity to these two fruits irritated her bladder.

Children's allergic reactions to foods are often very intense. One boy was so allergic to his favorite food, turkey, that he could not be in the house when it was cooking. Even the odor of turkey would set him to wheezing. Nor could he return to the house until it had been aired.

Parents with hyperactive children or children with learning disabilities should investigate the strong possibility of allergy. One little girl was a puzzle to her parents and teachers because her abilities ebbed and flowed like the tide. One time she could read and the next time she could not. She was found to be reacting strongly to wheat, string beans, corn, tomatoes, milk, and apples. After five months of treatment with food shots, her scholastic standing was much improved.

Parents only aggravate the problem when they become annoyed at the irritability of their children, who just might be reacting to a food or chemical. Also, parents are doing their children great harm if they permit them to eat junk foods, laden with sugar and excitants in the form of additives and preservatives.

It is a sad commentary on modern child rearing that parents think they are depriving their children when they don't let them have junk foods. Early childhood is the time to establish healthy eating habits; if a child hasn't been exposed to junk foods and sweets, he won't develop cravings for them.

It is believed that parents can prevent addiction to various foods by not serving the same food more than once or twice a week and by not permitting the child to have the same special treat every day.

Dr. Joseph Morgan, a pediatric allergist, maintains that there would probably be no food allergies at all if we started infants on rotary diversified diets, omitting sugar and additives.[3] A rotary diversified diet is one which rotates and varies the foods (see Chapter 8). The underlying principle of this type of diet is that allergies and addiction are caused not so much by the quantity of food but by the frequency with which foods are eaten.

With his first solids, the child would learn to enjoy one food at a time and no food would be repeated at too-frequent intervals. Dr. Morgan feels that the child would also benefit if during pregnancy, his mother had a controlled, diversified diet and then breast-fed the baby the first year.

It is gratifying that mothers are becoming aware of the importance of breast-feeding babies. Unfortunately, many of these same mothers are not aware that they themselves should be eating pure foods. If they are going to be drinking cow's milk that is contaminated with insecticide or contains antibiotics or hormones, the baby will be ingesting these substances. The only way a mother's milk can be pure is if her diet is pure.

A highly toxic mother gave birth to a toxic child. The mother's diet was changed to one consisting only of pure foods. The breast-fed infant continued to have difficulty until they removed from the mother's diet the foods that the child reacted to. This seriously curtailed the mother's diet because the mother and the child were allergic to different foods.

It has long been suspected that a pregnant woman might abort if exposed to paint and similar products. Therefore, it is recommended that if a pregnant woman must paint, it should be in a well-ventilated room. What has not been widely recognized is that the pregnant woman's inhaling of toxic substances from paint products can affect the fetus. A classic case involves a family that we shall call the Johnsons.

In the fall of 1970 Dr. Randolph diagnosed a husband, wife, and college-age daughter as having chemical sensitivities. Because all the family liked arts and crafts, their home was permeated with chemical pollutants. The husband worked in graphics and did oil painting at home for recreation. Their symptoms in varying degrees were arthritic pains, dizzy spells, irritability, inability to concentrate or make decisions, gastrointestinal problems, and lack of muscular coordination.

Through trial and error, making many mistakes along the way, they set about allergy-proofing their home following the procedures that will be outlined further along in the book. As a result of all this care, the Johnson family enjoys better health seven years later. The daughter managed to graduate from a local college by commuting and returning at night to the completely pure environment of her home. She even received a second college degree, in music. This was remarkable because her poor muscular coordination had previously made it impossible for her to continue playing the piano. Depression and inability to concentrate had also interfered with college course work and daily living.

The most important point, though, is that the illness of the child might have been avoided had Mrs. Johnson understood that no product is safe for everyone. When Mrs. Johnson was seven months pregnant with her daughter, she had set about fixing up the nursery for the baby and had painted a chest of drawers. She had followed the directions to the letter, taking all necessary precautions. Then, not liking the color, she had applied paint remover, again following the directions to the letter.

She was rushed to the hospital with a case of toxemia, and for two-and-a-half months, they were not sure if she and the baby would survive. They made it, but both are now considered chemical victims for life.

It is especially sad that the child became the victim of her mother's mistakes. Looking back, Mrs. Johnson realizes that she did three things which injured her child. First, she smoked cigarettes; second, she used paint with injurious fumes; and third, she inhaled the injurious fumes of paint remover.

"All this could have been prevented," said Mrs. Johnson sadly, "had I but known."

CHAPTER 4

Troublemakers at Home and at Work

IT SEEMS that whichever way we turn we are swallowing or touching or breathing things that produce stress. Clinical ecologists point out that modern chemicals are the most stress-producing factors of our environment. And our food itself breaks down into chemicals which may be hard on the human body. For example, ethanol (alcohol) is found in some fruits; phenols are common in plants and in milk; ethylene occurs in apples. What makes the load harder to bear is that other chemicals such as insecticides, flavorings, artificial colorings, and preservatives are added to the food in varying degrees.

Dr. Iris Bell puts it well: "For the person who is susceptible to ecologic illness, every meal adds a sizable load of natural and artificial chemicals which, taken together, require a great deal of adaptation by the body." She cites as one small example the innocent-seeming cornflakes we have for breakfast, which load the body up not only with corn, sugar, malt, artificial vitamins, and salt but also hydroxytoluene, BHA, and BHT. These latter are butylated hydroxyanisole and butylated hydroxytoluene, which are preservatives and solvents.

It goes without saying that the body takes a beating as it tries to adapt to too many foods that are loaded with added chemicals.

The air we breathe has its own array of added chemicals and can cause complaints ranging from mild to severe, from smarting eyes to poor vision, from stuffy noses to disabling asthma, from a mild circulatory problem to life-threatening cardiovascular disease, from mild mental confusion to serious mental disorders.

Later in the chapter we shall present a list of common troublemakers found in most homes. But first, let's consider some easy changes.

A major problem is a lack of knowledge on the part of the public, due primarily to the power of advertising. A good example is what we wear. The public was "educated" about the "advantage" and convenience of drip-dry fabrics. The demand for no-iron fabrics became so great that companies competed for stronger formulas for materials that needed no ironing and no dry cleaning. After nylon, a mildly toxic substance made from plastic, manufacturers moved to Dacron and

Orlon, which are even more toxic. Then they discovered polyester, which is probably the most toxic of all.

Although numerous articles have been written about the dangers of these toxins, people tend to ignore them. Intelligent people will say, "What are we supposed to do? Give up all of these conveniences?" What they don't realize is that so many of the chronic illnesses discussed in Chapter 1 are really the hidden dangers of the here and now.

But not everyone is ready to make drastic changes. With that in mind, we can only recommend that you avoid the most toxic products. By selective and informed purchasing, you will find that your life style does not have to change greatly. It will be well worth your time and effort to reduce the contaminants in your environment.

It is unfortunately true that any synthetic can be a source of trouble. You should avoid purchasing plastic items, for example. There are many products that are—or contain—plastics but we do not think of them as such. Both soft and hard plastics are contaminants. Some give off more contaminants when heated, as in the case of Bakelite handles on pots and pans.

People think that a plastic shower curtain, while it has an offensive smell when new, becomes tolerable after a few days. They assume that, because the odor has diminished, the chemical fumes have diminished as well. This is not necessarily the entire answer. What may have happened is that your body has adjusted to the fumes, and possibly at great cost.

Francis Silver, who serves as engineering consultant to the Society of Clinical Ecology, says that when you are exposed to the odor of rotten eggs a condition called "olfactory fatigue" sets in, so that the second breath smells only half as bad as the first. In other words, this fatigue has set in so quickly that your capacity for smelling has been diminished—but your vulnerability has not.

According to Silver, we absorb not only through the nose but by "inhaling" through the skin. A combination of the two causes a more serious and/or more lasting reaction, such as fatigue, backache, headache, irritability, a burning sensation under the skin. This inhaling through the skin can be compared with the body process involved when you have eaten garlic in substantial quantity and find that your skin gives off the odor of garlic. Your skin is in effect "exhaling."

Whether or not you can detect the injurious fumes in the environment, they are taking their toll. As for avoiding these pollutants, the acutely ill have no choice. At great cost, they must avoid everything that makes them ill. People with mild allergies and/or sensitivity to toxic products have a clear choice: simple preventive measures now or possibly drastic measures later. In either case, the rule of thumb should be that the treatment not be worse than the disease. The transition can be at your own pace, as long as you recognize that there is preventive value in acting sooner rather than later.

Immediate Changes. Find substitutes for toxic products which are frequently replenished. For example:

1. Discontinue buying anything in an aerosol can. (Use the more conventional container.)
2. Avoid highly perfumed petroleum-base cosmetics and toiletries. (Use unscented cosmetics or those made with natural herb scents.)
3. Avoid scented, tinted toilet paper, paper towels, facial tissues, etc. (Use pure, white, unscented products.)

Future Replacements. When purchasing durable goods, select products with the least amount of toxic materials. For example:

1. Avoid buying pots or pans of aluminum or with Teflon coating. Corningware and porcelain or enamel baked on cast iron are recommended. When possible, avoid Bakelite handles.
2. For redecorating or building a house, choose nontoxic furnishings, upholstery, paints, construction materials, etc., many of which are less costly than similar products that are toxic.
3. When buying clothes, avoid the most toxic materials such as polyester, and woolens which have been treated with dieldrin (mothproofing).

Simple Substitutes. So many products today cause needless pollution of the environment. Look for substitutes, such as:

1. To keep food warm, use an electric hot tray instead of a chafing dish heated by a Sterno flame or a candle.
2. As an all-purpose cleaner, use vinegar instead of a toxic cleaner such as ammonia or ammoniated products like Windex.
3. For laundering, use Borax and soap instead of bleach and detergents.
4. For table decorations, use flowers, fruits, or vegetables. If you must use candles, buy those made of beeswax.

(For a comprehensive list of the worst troublemakers, see Chapter 17).

For a handy reference, here is a list of troublemakers you might find in your own home.

TROUBLEMAKERS IN THE HOME

Aerosols	Car exhaust fumes entering the house
Air deodorizers, sprays	from an open window or an
Aluminum pots and pans	attached garage
Ammonia	Cedar-lined closets
	Charcoal
Bleaches	Chlorinated or fluoridated water

Christmas tree needles (which
  contain resin)
Cosmetics

Deodorants, anti-perspirants
Detergents
Disinfectants
Dyes

Electric blankets (because of plastic
  wires)

Felt-tip pens
Flameproof mattresses
Floor cleaners and waxes
Food additives
Fungicide-treated wallpaper
Furniture polish

Gas stoves and other gas appliances

Hair sprays
Heat-sealed soft plastic packages

Insecticide sprays and no-pest strips

Kerosene

Lacquer

Medications
Mineral oil
Mothballs and moth crystals
Mothproofed shelf paper
Mouthwash

Nail polish
Newspaper print (inks and solvents)

Oils for fans, sewing machines, etc.
Oven cleaner

Paint fumes
Paraffin
Perfumes, aftershaves
Permanent-press clothing
Pesticides
Pillowcases and sheets of synthetics
Pine-scented cleaners
Plastics (mattress covers, tablecloths,
  shower curtains, draperies, usually
  vinyl, food wrappers, shelf paper)

Refrigerant gas (check for leaks)
Rubber-backed carpets
Rubbing alcohol

Scented soaps
Shampoos
Soft plastic food containers and
  wraps
Solvents used for duplicating
  machines
Smoke from frying foods
Sponge rubber (mattresses and
  upholstery)
Stainproof upholstery and carpets
Synthetic clothing

Teflon pots and pans
Tin cans with phenol lining
Tobacco smoke
Toothpaste
Turpentine

Varnishes containing pesticides
Varsol

The fact that this is only a partial list indicates a need for more ecologic consultants like Francis Silver. It is interesting to see how Silver became involved in clinical ecology. Working in aircraft plants as an engineer, Silver first had his health impaired in 1956 from coal smoke and again in 1957 from tar fumes. His physical condition changed from rugged good health and no particular sensitivity to chronic illness and supersensitivity.

In his effort to lower his exposure to chemicals and so recover his health, he developed many techniques for diagnosing and eliminating problems of chemical exposure in the home and work environment. He became a sleuth. In 1962 Drs. Theron Randolph, Eloise Kailin, and Clifton Brooks launched him into this new endeavor in a formal way by referring some of their patients to him for consultation if they suspected the patient had a serious chemical problem in his home or place of work.

Francis Silver says it is his hope that this approach will be developed into a recognized profession so that each community will have some experts in the field.

Safety Hot Line. To report a product hazard or a product-related injury, call the U.S. Consumer Product Safety Commission, Washington, D.C., on the toll-free safety hot line 800-638-2666.

CHAPTER 5

Ecological Mental Illness

HERE IS a psychiatric case that reads like a mystery story. It's about a woman named Rhoda, who had been going to a psychiatrist for fifteen years. Instead of getting better, she grew steadily worse and kept increasing the frequency of her visits to the psychiatrist until she was going daily.

She was labeled neurotic and says she was told by the doctor that she was suffering from megalomania. Hoping to bolster her spirits, she began to redecorate her kitchen. At this point she became critically ill, began losing weight and having nightmares. The tranquilizers she was taking did nothing to deaden the pain in the left side of her neck or alleviate the depression which made her feel, she said, "as if the world were coming to an end."

Rhoda could scarcely eat anything, and experienced pain in the area of the colon accompanied by frequent nausea. Whenever she entered her kitchen she thought, "What an awful smell. It makes me sick to work in this kitchen!" She became overwhelmed with her work; the doctor assumed it was a reaction to her homemaking responsibilities.

Next she began avoiding the piano in the living room. Playing the piano had been a favorite form of relaxation for her. But "something about the living room bothered me," she said.

By now Rhoda was becoming suicidal and planned to slash her wrist—the left one, since it was the left side of her body that pained her the most. The pains moved to her legs, arms, and fingers. One doctor told her he could see that she had arthritis in her fingers.

Eventually she became so crippled she could hardly walk. Sometimes she couldn't tie her shoelaces. And there were times she had great difficulty getting out of bed. When she did manage to get out of bed, she held on to the walls for support. Gastro-intestinal tests to aid in diagnosing the colon problem revealed nothing.

The next difficulty that cropped up for Rhoda was mental confusion and inability to read.

Finally, her husband took issue with the psychiatrist who was suggesting that Rhoda's condition was psychosomatic.

Rhoda's husband came upon an article that led him to a clinical ecologist who suggested that Rhoda be taken to Dr. Randolph in Chicago. Rhoda arrived in Dr. Randolph's office in a wheelchair. He had her admitted to an ecologic unit of a hospital. On her first day in that pure environment, Rhoda was able to get out of her wheelchair.

As is the case with so many chemical victims, by the time Rhoda learned of her problem, she was already overloaded.

Francis Silver, the ecological engineer, visited her home and solved the mystery of the two rooms that were a particular problem to her. Where earlier it might have been thought that her avoidance of the kitchen related to some hidden aversion to kitchen duties or her avoiding the piano to some hidden need to avoid the discipline of piano practice, it now became apparent that the problem had indeed involved something hidden—hidden allergies.

Among other things, Rhoda was sensitive to the mustard gas in the glue of the new living-room wallpaper. The problem in the kitchen was the paints and solvents used in refinishing the cabinets.

It was determined that there were too many excitants in her home for Rhoda to return to good health, that it would be better to build a new house. Taking advantage of everything known to modern technology about purifying the air and eliminating pollutants, the new house contains only materials and products she can tolerate. And, of course, the excitants had to be removed from her diet as well; she was placed on a special rotation diet of organic foods.

As a result of living in her uncontaminated house, her appetite returned and Rhoda went back up to 110 pounds from the 90 pounds she had shrunk to. Gone are the arthritic pains and the depression. Not only is she tying her own shoelaces, but she is doing her own housework and enjoying it. She is also working long hours at their farm, where they are growing organic foods.

There was an exciting bonus for Rhoda and her husband involving their twelve-year-old daughter Jill, an allergic child who suffered severe asthmatic attacks requiring frequent hospital treatment. Jill was so impressed with the good results her mother achieved by following the rotary diet that she wondered if perhaps it might help her too. Jill began eating only organic foods on a rotation basis. The emergency trips to the hospital ceased. Jill's condition continues to improve.

When you think of Rhoda's long, wasted years of mistaken need for psychiatric treatment it makes you wonder: Why isn't it routine practice to test all psychiatric patients for environmental causes, when there are so many cases showing a definite relation between adverse environmental conditions and schizophrenia, manic depression, and other mental disorders?

The unaware physician should be made aware. The news media need to be educated as well. For example, research was incomplete for a program presented on television on May 26, 1977, entitled "Madness and Medicine," which was advertised as "Three key modes of treatment for the mentally ill: drugs, electric shock, and psychosurgery." Part of the program was devoted to former patients who revealed side effects from the therapy. Anyone who saw the program had to be moved by the statements made by these people who had been injured by their treatment—frequently administered without their permission.

The controversy over psychosurgery (brain surgery used in the treatment of certain mental disturbances) was discussed at length, and even the advocates labeled it as a "last resort." How can they call it a last resort when no mention was made of two methods of treatment that have been proven successful for countless patients who had previously been treated unsuccessfully? No mention was made of neuroallergy (allergy as it relates to the nervous system), one type of allergy discussed in this book, or orthomolecular psychiatry. The latter is practiced by many highly qualified, board-certified psychiatrists who take into consideration the part played by nutrition in mental health and who are concerned with such things as allergies and/or mineral and vitamin deficiencies.

As defined in California law, orthomolecular medicine is "the preservation of good health as well as the treatment of disease by providing the optimum molecular environment in the human body by varying the concentration in the body of vitamins, minerals, and other nutritional substances normally present in the body and required for health, and to include human ecology medicine which means discharge or avoidance of substances that are toxic or allergy-inducing to some patients."

You will notice that this definition includes "human ecology medicine." This is included thanks to the efforts and open-mindedness of Dr. David Hawkins, chairman of the Academy of Orthomolecular Psychiatry, and many of his colleagues, including a leader in his field, Dr. Carl Pfeiffer.[1] These psychiatrists are recognizing the need to remove the causes of psychiatric disorders rather than merely giving treatment. Many of them are referring patients to clinical ecologists. Others, like Dr. Karl Humiston of Sulphur Spring, Arkansas, Dr. Dale Peters of Wichita, Kansas, and Dr. Richard MacKarness of Basingstoke, England, have turned to clinical ecology, expanding their practices to include environmental control and dietary management.

Let us sidetrack for just a moment and tell you how a leading orthomolecular psychiatrist decided to add human ecology medicine to his practice.

"When I heard about cerebral allergy," he said, "I was sort of dubious. Then I heard some tapes of patients during their testing, and I said, 'Well, it could be.' When I saw movies of cases in a doctor's office, I was convinced. But it was my own personal experience that was the last piece of evidence that I needed.

"I developed diverticulitis and had to stop drinking milk. The first thing I noticed was that the incidence of my migraines dropped down to a quarter of what they used to be. I still had migraines on certain days, however.

"The next thing that happened was the real clincher. I had built a new house. Because it had been closed up, moths and other insects had invaded the place and I wanted to exterminate before moving in. Because the exterminator asked too high a price, I bought a gallon of commercial insecticide and started to spray it around the closets myself. Within a couple of minutes I got a headache that was just blinding. I recognized it as the same type of headache I developed periodically at the hospital. It turned out that the hospital was using the same kind of insecticide. When they discontinued using that insecticide, my headaches disappeared.

"That's when I thought to myself, 'If milk can lay me out for a couple of days with bad migraine, and if exposure to insecticide can do the same thing, then what the clinical ecologists are saying must be true.' "

It's hard for the average person to believe that even hallucinations can be caused by foods. Dr. Iris Bell discussed this in a paper presented to the Tenth Advanced Seminar in Clinical Ecology, Dallas, Texas.[2] Dr. Bell at that time was engaged in research at the Department of Psychiatry and Behavior Sciences, Stanford University Medical Center. She reported the case of a thirty-nine-year-old narcoleptic whose symptoms "ranged from excessive daytime sleepiness, sleep attacks and fatigue, depression, and visual hallucinations, to chronic diarrhea, headaches, thirst and episodic gastrointestinal bleeding. . . . At one point he was taking up to forty different pills to control his symptoms."

He showed marked improvement from ecologic treatment. However, "an accidental exposure to the odor of dish detergent brought such a reaction of irritability that he physically attacked his two sons.

"The dish-detergent reaction with the symptoms of irritability and aggression was one of the clues in my observations of ecology patients over the past several years which have led me to hypothesize that the olfactory system of the central nervous system (CNS) is directly involved in the mechanisms of ecologic mental illness."

According to Dr. Bell, odors have ready access to the brain: "Once odor triggers a particular response in the olfactory bulb neurons, the firing of these cells can directly influence the function of a wide variety of central nervous system reactions. It might be speculated that specific odors could excessively stimulate or depress certain circuits to produce the manic-depressive swings of mood seen in some ecologic patients."

It is especially sad when a child is diagnosed as having a mental illness when he or she is really the victim of severe allergies. Such was the case of C.S., a ten-year-old girl; when she was tested with petro-chemical ethyl alcohol (ethanol), she reacted with complete irrationality for three hours, screaming, biting, and becoming hyperactive.[3] She also regressed to infantile behavior and was so disoriented that she no longer recognized her mother, who was sitting next to her. She thought her mother was "a former male teacher whose class she had been in two years previously."

Asked to count, C.S. gave numbers out of sequence and confused them with some of the letters of the alphabet. She thought she saw purple things floating in the air and thought marking pencils were carrots. She could not remember where she lived.

After the ethanol wore off she could not remember the symptoms she had just experienced.

That was C.S.'s reaction in a clinical test. But every day of her life had been a nightmare of its own. It was found that natural gas in the kitchen stove of her house often caused her to stagger. The fumes from automobiles affected her and she once walked into the side of a car. The solvent xylene, from a felt-tip marker, caused headaches, blurred vision, and irritability. She once became so irritated when using a felt-tip marker in art class that she deliberately destroyed the poster she had been drawing.

Such bizarre behavior in the past has labeled a child "incorrigible" or "mentally sick," but enlightened doctors and psychiatrists are finally coming to see that the trouble may lie in the environment or diet and not in the child.

Sometimes the incidents of clinical ecologic illness diagnosed as mental disorders result in advice that could not be more harmful. One woman had been told by her psychiatrist that her severe emotional problems involving her mother were causing her to have an attack of asthma whenever she was in the kitchen and the stove was on. Her family encouraged her to stay in the kitchen as much as possible to "confront and overcome her feelings." Eventually, testing showed that she was sensitive to gas and had a chemical susceptibility to various petroleum compounds. The gas, not her mother, was her problem.

Some people mistakenly equate alcoholism with emotional disorders. Tom J., labeled an alcoholic, had been going to a psychiatrist for over a year and was told he was emotionally immature because he became tense and full of anxiety that bordered on panic. As it turned out, he was sensitive to brewer's yeast and the fermented sugars in the grains and fruits from which alcoholic beverages are made. The psychiatrist had not understood his problem at all. (Not only was Tom allergic to yeast, but also to molds and to the grains from which alcohol is made—corn, wheat, and rye—even in the form of cereals and breads.)

Very often the real problem of alcoholism is an addiction to the grain in the beverage. In such a person, eating corn can provoke a craving not only for corn but for bourbon and other alcoholic beverages.

Once again we must raise the question, Why isn't something being done about this? How frustrating it is that no one seems to be getting the message across to alcoholics and their families.

Many problems of children traditionally labeled mental or emotional disorders—such as autism, hyperactivity, learning disabilities—have been found to result from exposure to pollutants. If this book accomplishes nothing else, we hope it will alert parents to the need for consultation with a clinical ecologist to evaluate the possibility.

Not only parents need to be made aware of the behavioral effects from exposure to allergens. Penal authorities need to be alerted as well. There is some evidence that allergies may be implicated in our high crime rate. Dr. Humiston has been interested in the study of criminals and their reactions to foods.

One study involved an alleged bank robber. The court had ordered a pre-trial evaluation because "although he had spent ten of the past twenty years serving three sentences in prison, it appeared that this offense was part of a distinct pattern of deterioration in his mental and physical functioning."

In food tests administered after therapeutic fasting, the subject developed immediate strong allergic reactions to most of the sixty foods tested as well as to chlorinated water and hydrocarbon chemicals. To quote Dr. Humiston, "His main reactions to foods were to become depressed and hostile, sometimes after an initial stimulatory 'high.' "

These are just a few of the results: "The angry-hostile reactions followed wheat, peanuts, rye, cheddar cheese, lentil, cashew, pork, molasses, perch, canned tuna, canned peach, beef and corn. He acted out hostility by throwing or breaking things after beef and corn. He became very moody and depressed following beef, honey, orange, wheat, yeast, cod, perch, strawberry and raisin."

The encouraging thing is that after going on a prescribed diet the subject felt so vastly improved that he no longer felt stuck in his behavioral rut. Dr. Humiston described it, "For the first time in twenty years the man was able to picture himself as a non-criminal."

"I am a different person," he told Dr. Humiston.

CHAPTER 6

Allergies and Heart Disease

THEY USED to call it acute indigestion. Then they labeled it heart attack. Now there is increasing evidence that perhaps they were right in the first place. Very often it is a digestive reaction to a food or chemical excitant—a causal agent—which, when severe enough, triggers a heart attack.

It is not always easy to diagnose. For example, William, a man in his late thirties, took his wife to a clinical ecologist for testing. During the course of the conversation with the doctor, he mentioned that while his wife had allergy problems he did not. His problem was a heart condition that was difficult to diagnose. Following each attack hospital tests showed no damage to his heart.

As a result of his conversation with the doctor, William decided to be tested for possible food allergies. His reaction to milk was symptomatic of a heart attack. Since abstaining from milk products, he has had no further incidence.

Sometimes it is more than just foods; chemicals frequently are the causative agents. An example of a more extreme case is that of Dr. C., who had spent several hours making duplicating machine copies, after which he ate a meal containing food to which he was sensitive. He then suffered a heart attack.

Knowing that he was food-sensitive, he got in touch with a cardiovascular surgeon who was on the staff of a hospital with an ecologic unit. Here Dr. C. was tested for food and chemical sensitivities. Each time a test was given for a food or chemical to which he was sensitive, heart irregularity resulted, confirming the suspicion that the heart attack was precipitated by the overloading of food and chemical excitants. He is now functioning normally as long as he exercises caution with his diet and his environment.

There are other vascular disorders related to allergies. A good example is the case of Howard, a twenty-eight-year-old man who had recurring phlebitis. He developed several blood clots in his lungs, and his legs were affected to the point where he was unable to walk. None of the customary medication helped him. He was brought into a hospital ecologic unit and fasted for five days, after which the phlebitis symptoms disappeared.

When Howard was tested for fumes from natural gas, within a few minutes he again experienced the pain that accompanies phlebitis. Similar reactions occurred after his tests for perfumes, detergents, and several foods. Since that time he has avoided the excitants that cause the condition and has not required medication. He has had recurrence of the ailment only when he has been overexposed.

Reynaud's disease is another vascular disorder that warrants this ecologic approach; the patient should be checked for allergies and sensitivities. Marian, a young woman, was bothered by extreme sensitivity to cold. She went to a doctor because, among other things, her fingers had a tendency to turn blue. Her problem was diagnosed as Reynaud's disease, a circulatory illness. The doctor prescribed several medications to thin her blood and dilate her blood vessels. After taking the medication for a few days she developed severe headaches. Her doctor then prescribed medication for the headaches so that she could continue to take vasodilators—drugs that dilate blood vessels. Nothing seemed to help.

To prevent the progression of gangrene and the necessity of amputating the finger, which had turned black, the doctor suggested clipping some of the nerves that regulate the tone of the blood vessels. Marian asked for a consultation and was directed to a cardiovascular surgeon who admitted her to an ecologic unit. By the time she reached the unit, the black finger had become ulcerated. The condition was so advanced that it was suspected that the finger would indeed have to be amputated.

After she spent a few days in the unit, the blood started circulating through the fingers, the ulcerations began to clear up, and the finger was saved. It was subsequently discovered that the cause of the poor circulation was sensitivity to certain foods as well as to chemicals. Now, by avoiding these excitants she prevents the symptoms of Reynaud's disease. If she is exposed to the excitants, she suffers a recurrence of the symptoms.

During her interview at the ecologic unit it was learned that she had a family history of vascular illness. Her paternal great-grandmother had died of a stroke at thirty-seven; her grandmother, at thirty-nine; her father, at forty; and his brother, at forty-three. Marian recalled her father's symptoms: spontaneous breathing difficulty, numbness in his arms, swelling of his lips (which increased whenever he ate certain foods). He would be hospitalized and tested for heart involvement and each time the test results were negative. Yet he died of cerebral hemorrhage at forty.

In the light of her own experience, Marian now realizes that her father's circulatory illness could have resulted from exposure to chemicals. Although it can't be proved that this was so, she recalls that he was unable to tolerate many chemical products and had frequent asthmatic attacks. This leads her to believe that she and her father suffered from the same problem, food and chemical sensitivities.

Today there is increasing evidence that environmental control and proper diet can prevent some of the heart surgery being performed. Karen, a young woman in her late thirties worked with her father in his laboratory and lived in the apartment above. She had been ill for some time, had had four coronary artery bypasses, and still suffered chest pains and heart irregularities. After surgery failed to improve her condition, it was suggested that she enter a hospital ecologic unit.

Karen's condition improved even though all medication was discontinued; the chest pain and heart irregularities disappeared. Following a prescribed procedure she was tested first for foods and then for chemicals. After her test for beef, her chest pains and irregular heartbeat returned. When she was tested for formaldehyde and other chemicals she had the same reaction.

By the end of the testing period, it was concluded that because she had always lived above a laboratory, inhaling fumes such as formaldehyde, and had always worked with these chemicals, she could no longer tolerate them. As is frequently the case with many severely allergic patients, her chemical sensitivities spilled over into an intolerance not only to the beef but to other foods as well.

Another example showing how dangerous toxic chemicals can be is that of a young concert harpist whose career was brought to an abrupt halt when she developed paralysis on the right side of her body. When she was tested for rabbit or wheat, her breathing stopped. In addition to these allergies it was learned that she was allergic to plastic. After a bit of detective work, it was discovered that during the course of bladder repair surgery, plastic mesh had been used. She was taken to surgery where the plastic mesh was removed. As a result the paralysis disappeared, and her career has resumed again with promise of great success. This case brings into question the safety of intrauterine devices, silicone implantation, and false teeth or caps made of plastic.

You can see from the variety of these cases that there is a correlation between sensitivity to excitants and cardiovascular diseases. All heart specialists, and in fact many laymen, are aware of the environmental factors relating to heart trouble. Every time there is a pollution alert they advise heart patients to take precautions. The difference between most physicians and those practicing clinical ecology is that the latter test the direct cause and effect of the disease and treat accordingly.

Once again we remind you that it is not our intention to state categorically that all illnesses are allergy-related or induced. However, any illness that goes undiagnosed might benefit from the attention of a clinical ecologist. Chemical intolerance is insidious because chemicals are absorbed by the skin through osmosis. The chemicals are, so to speak, inhaled into every part of your body, entering the bloodstream. Other inhalants such as molds and dust also enter the bloodstream, as do the foods we eat. That's why it bears repeating that disease of any tissue, organ or body system can be affected by allergies to food, drugs, chemicals, and other inhalants.

CHAPTER 7

Stress Reduction

MANY EMINENT medical researchers such as Dr. Hans Selye (author of *The Stress of Life*) have proven in repeated laboratory experiments that stress can cause ulcers, heart conditions, and many other serious physical ailments.[1]

There are some excellent books dealing with stress: the dangers of stress, how to avoid it, how to reduce it. To most of us, stress means tension resulting from a quarrel with a loved one, an unpleasant disagreement with an employer, a near-collision with another automobile, the loss of a job.

Now clinical ecologists are telling us that our bodies suffer harmful consequences when we are exposed to stress caused by toxic chemicals that are present in the air we breathe, the water we drink, and the food we eat. The body functions can be damaged severely by the substances that man has introduced into the environment: the concoctions of his brain that are foreign to his body.

"Stress is a pressure," Dr. Karl Humiston explains. "It can be literal physical pressure, or pressure from situations, people, foods, chemicals, allergies, or our own struggles.

"Within healthy limits, stress stimulates healthy responses, and is a necessity of life. Beyond these limits, stress can prevent healthy functioning, at times to the point of endangering life. Healthy limits vary, depending on your state of functioning at the time.

"The normal processing of incoming food, in a healthy state, is a heavy load, just as carrying a ton of potatoes is a heavy load for a truck. It is a load for which we are designed, and therefore, it is a healthy stress.

"The processing of foods to which we are allergic, or of synthetic chemicals for which we have no natural enzymes, is an unhealthy stress. The healthy stress will stimulate our normal energy, and the latter will make us sick. The sick person's system needs to rest for a while. For the mildly allergic, stress reduction is advisable; for those with severe allergies, it is mandatory."

Clinical ecologists say that the major way to deal with stress and restore the body to a healthy state is by avoiding the causes—in other words, environmental control. We are in total agreement. To expand on that approach, and as a result of our personal experience, the procedures set forth in the following pages are recommended as an addition to—not a substitute for—environmental control and proper diet.

This chapter should not be interpreted as a shortcut to restored health; it is intended as an aid. There are no shortcuts, and those who rely on get-well-quick methods will find they aggravate instead of improve their condition.

The procedures described in this chapter will show you how to reduce stress. The suggestions will expand your capacity to handle life's experiences with less stress, rather than suggesting any reduction in your activities.

All aspects of living provide a degree of stress; eating, drinking, exercising, sexual intercourse—living is stress. The object is to learn which are the unavoidable unhealthy stresses and how to deal with them. The effects of stress can be diminished by the way we handle it; by learning to work with our bodies through proper exercise, proper breathing, proper relaxation techniques.

LEARNING TO BREATHE PROPERLY

Almost everyone is born with the ability to breathe properly. However, as children we are scolded and told to "stand up straight, pull in your tummy, throw out your chest," all of which can develop unhealthy breathing habits. The mind takes over and unknowingly controls what is supposed to be involuntary, the autonomic system with functions such as the beating of the heart, circulation of the blood, and breathing.

Many therapists believe that the inability to handle stress as an adult is a result of the manner in which they as children escape from unhappy feelings by cutting off their breathing. For example, a young child frequently will "turn blue" when frustrated. What is actually happening is that he has restricted his breathing. That pattern, built up over a period of years, leads to bad breathing habits.

There is an important childhood ability that we have lost. That is the power to let grief "flow." When a young child is hurt physically, he cries. If his feelings are hurt, he cries. If he is humiliated, he cries. Frank Silver, who has studied the effects of grief, says:

"It appears that the 'flow' of grief must be a universal healing mechanism for both physical and mental hurt or pain . . . like the surging and ebbing tide, cleansing and soothing . . .

"If a child who has been hurt is encouraged to cry out an injury completely, he starts laughing and then runs off to play again happily. How long this full healing may take depends upon the severity of the injury. With very severe injury, the crying may take quite a long time, even many hours.

"The human organism will use grief spontaneously to heal itself, unless taught not to. Laughter, yawning, talking and convulsive movements such as trembling or tantrum-like behavior are other forms of flow used in healing."

When the flow of grief is stifled, the child becomes tense, much like a frightened animal that senses danger. His breathing changes from the relaxed, natural rhythm to short, constricted breaths. Unfortunately, with each new unpleasant experience, he reinforces the poor breathing habit.

We have found two ways to test your breathing habits. First, check to see if you breathe properly:

Stand up. Place your hand on your abdomen; move your hand up as far as you can without touching the bone. The soft area just below your rib cage is your diaphragm.

Holding your hand on your diaphragm, inhale deeply and then exhale. Repeat several times. Notice the movement of your hand as you breathe. Does it move in as you inhale and out as you exhale? If so, you are breathing incorrectly.

Think of your diaphragm as a balloon being filled with air. As it fills up with air, it inflates; as it loses air, it deflates. Therefore, as your diaphragm fills up with air—inhaling—it should be expanding, pushing your hand out. As you exhale, your diaphragm should be deflating and your hand should be moving back into position. This is known as diaphragmatic breathing.

Next, check to see if you are controlling your breathing or if it is truly spontaneous. You will be lying down for this test, but before you do so, get a paper bag and have it handy in case you hyperventilate enough to cause tingling around the lips or spasms in the hands or feet. Should that happen, simply blow into the bag—as if you are blowing up a balloon—so that you can rebreathe your own carbon dioxide. There is no cause for alarm; divers sometimes have a similar problem of balancing the amount of oxygen and carbon dioxide they need.

Now lie down and *pant*—loud, rapid inhaling and exhaling, like the panting of a dog. Continue to pant until your breathing automatically switches over to a deep diaphragmatic breathing. If you have to help the changeover from panting to diaphragmatic breathing by swallowing, your breathing is controlled. You cannot reach your true depth of relaxation so long as you are controlling your breathing.

There are many systems which have the goal of teaching relaxation. Unfortunately, too many procedures teach breath *control*. It is our premise that the secret is not control but rather relinquishing control not only of our breathing, but of our entire autonomic or involuntary nervous system.

STRESS REDUCTION THERAPY

In an effort to find new ways to reduce stress, a group of chemically sensitive patients studied self-relaxation, meditation, massage, yoga, and other exercises taken from both Eastern and Western cultures.[2] We found some help in all systems. Combining some features of these techniques, we arrived at a new form of relaxation by self-suggestion. We learned to reach a level of relaxation so deep that we were able to relinquish control of the autonomic system in order to slow the pulse, lower or raise blood pressure, increase circulation, regulate the heartbeat, and so forth. In so doing, the individual is able to raise or lower the temperature in affected parts of the body, relieve or eliminate migraine headaches or migraine equivalent, lower the respiration rate, reduce or eliminate edema.

With this new procedure we found great help in reducing stress. Both when working by ourselves and with other allergy patients, we discovered that other procedures were sometimes counterproductive. For example, it is frequently recommended that the patient concentrate on directing warmth to an arm or leg by repeating the phrase "My right arm is heavy and warm, my right arm is heavy and warm." The patient who does not feel warmth could become frustrated and, if anything, experience greater stress. Unfortunately, there are many patients who do not feel the warmth initially. The problem stems from the assumption that everyone experiences the same sensations in a state of relaxation. Nothing could be further from the truth.

Here is one way to help people find their own state of relaxation. For the purposes of this program, we deal with three phases of the process called stress reduction therapy, a name suggested by Dr. James Parsons, a psychiatrist from Melbourne, Florida.

A word of advice before you begin. Don't take yourself too seriously. This is an exercise for reducing stress. Getting upset while trying to learn it would defeat the purpose. You may find it helpful to start by reading the description of the process, not once but two or three times.

That way you will understand the purpose and the goal of the procedure. Once you understand it, begin practicing. Keep practicing until you have reached the desired effect.

Don't be discouraged if it takes more time than you expected it to. The important thing is to give it a fair chance. You may find it encouraging to learn that when others had become proficient and were able to reach a level of total relaxation, they found the procedure serving in many instances as a substitute for medication. There are many cases in which stress reduction therapy has speeded the healing of open wounds, helped broken bones mend more quickly, prevented blistering after burns, and even cleared blurred vision.

At first sight, the procedures may appear difficult. However, if the instructions below are read carefully in their entirety before you begin, the exercise will no longer seem difficult.

1. Read, and if necessary reread, the detailed instructions until you are sure you understand what you are supposed to do.

2. Read the *abbreviated instructions* (page 67), making a mental note of each step.

3. Copy the abbreviated instructions onto a 3″ × 5″ card for easy reference so that you won't have to refer to the book while practicing.

4. Do not begin until you see the words "It is now time to begin to practice" written in CAPITAL LETTERS.

PHASE 1
HOW TO ACHIEVE THE RELAXED FEELING

Lie down in a quiet place. Close your eyes to shut out visual distractions. Loosen any tight clothing. Do not use a pillow. If your neck is uncomfortable, fold a towel two or three times and place it under your head.

1. **Legs.** Compare them to each other. How do they feel? Does one leg feel better than the other? How? How do they feel against the mattress? Make a mental note of any sensations you have in your legs.

2. **Panting.** From earlier in this chapter, you will recall that panting is loud, rapid inhaling and exhaling like the panting of a dog. Pretend that you are blowing up that balloon we spoke of before.

Place your hand on your diaphragm (the soft part below your rib cage). As you inhale, be sure that your hand is forced up; as you exhale, your hand falls back.

Continue to pant until your breathing switches over to automatic diaphragm breathing. If this does not happen automatically while you're learning, swallowing can help induce the change to diaphragm breathing. (In time, with enough practice, maybe weeks, maybe months, your body will perform this function automatically. Until then, you will always practice coordinating exhaling with relaxing as described in the next few paragraphs.)

3. **Relax right leg.** First, you must compare the sensations in your legs so that you will be able to make note of the difference between your left leg—which is not involved—and the right leg, which you are in the process of relaxing.

The premise here is that the best way to know when you are really relaxing is to have a basis for comparison. This comparison includes the procedure that involves tensing the muscles and relaxing them.

4. **Synchronize breathing.** Now you are ready to synchronize your breathing with what you are doing with your right leg. Breathe in as you tense your leg, breathe out as you relax your leg. When you relax the muscle, remember to do so slowly to avoid strain.

It is very important that all these instructions be followed exactly as described because the body will then, in most cases, condition itself to relax automatically every time you breathe out, even when you are not exercising.

5. **Stretch toes.** Lie flat so that your legs are full length. Without moving your leg, stretch the toes of your right foot toward your head and tense your right leg.

Compare the feeling in the right leg with the feeling in the left leg. See how long you have to tense up before you notice a distinct difference between the two legs.

Hold your breath as long as you can while you hold the tension in your right leg. Slowly breathe out and relax.

Don't release the tension in your leg too fast or it will be a strain on your muscles. Again, compare your legs to see at which point the right leg, with its tension, has returned to the state of the left leg, which has not been tensed, and what is more, at which point the right leg feels better and more relaxed as a result of the exercise. Repeat the procedure two or three times.

Give it a name. At this point, forget the word "relaxed" and develop a new, very personal language which defines your relaxed state. Be more specific. Instead of saying "more relaxed" or "less relaxed," say whether you feel warm or cool, heavy or light. Does your leg feel longer or shorter? Do you feel as if you are sinking or floating? Is there a tingling or sparking sensation? Is it energizing? Is it weightless?

You may be aware of a combination of these sensations. On the other hand, you may feel none of them. These are a few of the sensations that some people experience. Yours may be even more individualized, like the man who reported that his legs felt like huge watermelons.

The important thing is not to be influenced by what others feel. These examples are given to demonstrate what *you* are looking for.

A word of encouragement here, for persons who cannot detect any change at this point. Continue the rest of the exercise, following the instructions. There is no set pattern to determine who will eventually have the best results.

Some of the people who have benefited the most from this process felt nothing in the beginning. In fact, some at first felt a greater tightness, even discomfort. Now they achieve a state of such deep relaxation that they can, at will, anesthetize themselves, stop bleeding, and begin a process of speeding up the healing of wounds.

6. **Left leg.** Follow the same procedure as with the right leg.

7. **Both legs.** Now tighten both legs at the same time, following the same procedure you have been using with each leg individually. Note the continuing change in the sensations in your legs.

8. **Arms.** Proceed with your arms as you did with your legs. The one difference is that you apply the tension by making a fist with each hand.

Breathe in, make two fists, tense your arms as tightly as you can, creating enough tension so that it moves into your shoulders. Breathe out very, very slowly and relax. Repeat a couple of times until your arms are as relaxed as your legs.

9. **Jaws and face.** Pretend there is a pencil between your teeth. Bite down hard as if biting on the pencil, leaving a quarter-inch between your upper and lower teeth. As you breathe in, tighten your face, screw up your nose, and thrust your lower jaw forward, tensing all the muscles in your face, neck, and head. Slowly breathe out and relax.

10. **Torso.** As you breathe in, tighten your torso, the muscles in your abdomen, back, and buttocks. Tense your sphincter muscles. Slowly breathe out and relax.

11. **Finally, all parts together.** Now combine all the steps. Breathe in, tighten your whole body:

> Pull toes toward head . . . tighten legs.
> Make a fist . . . tighten arms and shoulders.
> Bite down . . . tighten face, head, and neck.
> Tighten abdomen, pelvis, buttocks.
> *Breathe out slowly . . . relax slowly . . . enjoy the release.*

12. **Enjoy.** Enjoy the relaxed state and be aware of your body, your breathing, your surroundings. You've earned the feeling of well-being that now floods through you.

Abbreviated Instructions

Before you begin to practice, copy the following abbreviated instructions onto a 3″ × 5″ card to have for easy reference on the bed beside your hand.

Inhale for tensing, exhale for relaxing.
Check body sensations between steps.

1. Lie down . . . close eyes . . . compare legs.
2. Tighten and relax:
     Right leg, left leg, both legs.
     Right arm, left arm, both arms.
     Jaws, face, head, neck.
     Upper and lower torso.
     Whole body.

Final Instructions

For your first attempt, allow an hour of quiet time, preferably before bedtime. (Gradually you will learn to accomplish the same results in just a few minutes in spite of any noise or commotion around you.)

Loosen your clothing. Place the card of abbreviated instructions on the bed within easy reach. Have a paper bag handy to blow into in case you hyperventilate.

IT IS NOW TIME TO BEGIN TO PRACTICE.

PHASE 2

To avoid confusion do not even read this phase until you have mastered Phase 1, so do practice every day.

You will know you have mastered Phase 1 when you experience a new sensation which from this point on will be referred to as *the feeling.* It is very individualistic. No one can describe it for you. When you get it, you will know.

To help you recognize *the feeling* at the end of Phase 1, be aware of your total sensation, how you feel on the mattress—if you feel it at all. How your arms feel—if you can feel them at all. In other words, take particular note of the sensation you most enjoy and of which you are most aware. Give it a name. For example, "this weightless feeling," "this floating feeling," "this heavy feeling," "this tingling feeling," "this energizing feeling," "this lack of feeling," or any other name that will identify your feeling of relaxation.

Don't adopt labels that you may have heard others use in referring to *their* relaxed feeling. Use the word or expression that best describes what *you* are feeling in the relaxed state.

Now that you have given a name to your feeling, use it freely in this phase, substituting it whenever you read the words *the feeling*. This new language is a way for you to communicate with your own body: "I feel weightless," or "I'm energized," or "I'm tingling," or "I have a heavy feeling."

Conditioning Process

Conditioning is the keystone of Phase 2. Psychology defines conditioning as a process by which a response comes to be elicited by a stimulus—a feeling, an object, a situation—to which one would not naturally or normally respond in that way. In other words, if you normally react in a given way, you can train yourself to react in the same way to a different stimulus, through the constant association of one with the other.

We believe that for the conditioning process to work in stress reduction, it is necessary for the subject to be totally convinced that he has the ability to help his physical condition by his thoughts.

The process that is being introduced here is not new. We were born with this ability but usually use it negatively. For example, an infant, in the presence of a mother who is very disturbed, picks up the mother's tension.

It is our belief that tensions can be transmitted to an area of one's anatomy. An infant can refer that tension to his skin, for example, resulting in eczema, or to his stomach in the form of colic, or to his liver in the form of toxicity in the system. In an adult, probably the most common manifestation of this negative transmission is the tension headache.

Stress of any kind transmitted to any part of the body results in numerous stress disorders. Working from this premise, we have studied stress reduction techniques to change these negative transmissions into positive results.

If negative thoughts can cause headaches, why can't positive thoughts prevent or erase them? The answer is, they can.

Combining these premises, we developed the following conditioning process to reinforce positive thoughts by repetition.

Read all the instructions first, as you did in Phase 1.

Do not begin to practice until you reach the end of the instructions and find the words "You may now begin this phase," written in CAPITAL LETTERS.

At the end of Phase 1, enjoying the sensation created by total relaxation, you gave the name to *the feeling* as described above. Now, as step one of Phase 2, you are ready to condition your body to return to your deepest level of relaxation which you now call *the feeling*.

Each time you work at this you will reach a different level of relaxation. Sometimes the state of relaxation is retarded because of pressures and tensions at the time you are practicing the procedure. This is particularly true if you are having a hay fever type reaction or an allergic reaction from a chemical exposure. That can be the worst type of stress. And, of course, the level of relaxation you reach is largely determined by the level of tension at which you began. Therefore, the fact that you do not achieve a deeper level of relaxation each time does not necessarily indicate that there has been no improvement in the technique or that you are not progressing.

The conditioning consists of breathing exercises, accompanied by specific thoughts. It involves breathing in as you count, and breathing out as you relax.

As you are breathing out and thinking "Relax into *the feeling*," it is important to conjure up *the feeling*. Slowly give your body time to respond, talk to yourself, telling yourself something like this:

"Now, as I lie here, if I really wish to learn to return to this level of relaxation in a matter of seconds, I must concentrate on *the feeling*. I am letting my body soak in *the feeling*. I am aware of *the feeling* penetrating my mind, my body, the very core of my being.

"I am talking to my body, saying to my body, 'My arms and legs are aware of *the feeling* . . . my torso is aware of *the feeling* . . . I sense *the feeling* in my head . . . I sense *the feeling* in my organs. *The feeling* penetrates every nerve in my body . . . every muscle in my body . . . every cell in my body.'

"As I go into a deeper and deeper state of relaxation, my body is conditioning itself to return to this state by using the formula."

FORMULA FOR PHASE 2

Breathing in Deeply	*Breathing out Slowly*
Think "one"	Relax into *the feeling*
Think "two"	Relax into *the feeling*
Think "three"	Relax into *the feeling*

Practice the formula two or three times, letting your body soak up *the feeling* into your consciousness so that you will be able to return to it at will.

Breathe in deeply, feeling the air expand your abdomen, your diaphragm, and all the way up into your chest, your back, and your shoulders. Then very slowly and lingeringly, breathe out, allowing yourself to relax into *the feeling* which you have experienced during your deepest state of relaxation.

For want of a better, more concise term, the formula states that you "think" *the feeling*. Obviously you can't "think" a feeling—more is involved than just experiencing it or being *aware* of it. What you are really doing is *training your body and your mind to register the feeling* so that the next time you can begin where you left off.

Today you begin where you left off yesterday. With today's process you relax more deeply, and then you condition yourself to begin tomorrow where you left off today.

It is an interesting cycle. People have reported that once they've reached a very deep level they have been unaware of a daily change. From time to time, maybe weeks in between, they are suddenly aware of an entirely new experience, a new tranquillity and peace of mind.

We and people we have trained use Phase 1 for half an hour a day, deepening the level so that the body will condition itself to be relaxed at its "norm," being tense only during traumas.

During the day, to reduce stress, apply the formula for Phase 2 for a three-minute period from time to time. That is a potent way for the body to condition itself to throw off needless tensions. In that way you can handle more stress without injury to your health, even the unavoidable unhealthy stress caused by indoor and outdoor pollution.

Continue the conditioning by thinking something like this:

"If I really wish to learn to return to this state in a matter of minutes, when I count back from three to zero, I shall be wide awake and alert, but so completely relaxed that the conditioning will have taken effect.

"When I count back from three to zero, I shall be wide awake and alert and so relaxed that my body will have absorbed *the feeling*.

"When I count back from three to zero, I shall be wide awake and alert but so completely relaxed that *the feeling* will have penetrated my mind as well as my body."

Now think to yourself:

"*Three*, back to normal, leaving all fantasies behind.

"*Two*, so completely relaxed that my mind, my body, my inner core is absorbing *the feeling*.

"*One*, conditioned to return to *the feeling* by using the formula.

"*Zero*, wide awake and alert, yet completely relaxed."

YOU ARE NOW READY TO BEGIN TO PRACTICE PHASE 2.

After you have completed Phase 2, get up, walk around, return to normal. After five or ten minutes, lie down again.

PHASE 3

Do not go on to this phase until you have practiced and mastered Phase 2.

Phase 3 begins five or ten minutes after completing Phase 2.

The object of Phase 3 is to test the conditioning process of Phase 2. Can you now return to *the feeling* you experienced at the end of Phase 1 without using the procedure of Phase 1 but by merely using the Phase 2 formula?

Phase 1 established *the feeling*.

Phase 2 starts with *the feeling* and conditions you to return to it with the formula.

Phase 3 tests the formula to see if you can return to *the feeling* just by using the formula.

If after three attempts it doesn't come easily, don't be discouraged. Turn in for the night and try again tomorrow. Remember, everyone is an individual. Some people need more conditioning than others. It may be that you are carrying a great deal of responsibility in your home life or job or it may be ragweed season and you are therefore subjected to an unusual amount of stress.

Ironically, it seems the people who need more time for the process· are those who don't have the time. Take it from those who know from sad experience, *it is worth taking the time*. Not only is it important for your state of health, but paradoxically, it will save you time. You will require less sleep because your sleep will be more restful. You will wake up more refreshed. You will have more energy during the day.

SUMMARY

Stress is a common ingredient in today's society. This chapter has described one method of minimizing its effects—the one that we found to be the most helpful to the greatest number of people. Obviously, there are other methods of relaxation. The important thing is to find the method that works best for you and practice it diligently.

If you can master a relaxation technique, you will be able to accomplish more in a given amount of time than ever before in your life.

PART II

DIET PLANNING

CHAPTER 8

The Rotary Diversified Diet

WE CONSIDER this chapter the one that will probably change your life more than any other in the book. To take you into a different world of diet—a totally different concept of meal planning—let us tell you about Billy Casper, well known in sports circles. He's the golfer who won the U.S. Open in 1959. But he was best known for his bad temper and big bay window. Over a twelve-year period his earnings were second only to Arnold Palmer's. But though he was a winner, he was avoided by fans and sportswriters alike, who couldn't take his crankiness, his insults and general irritability. Casper acted as if he didn't care what they thought. He seemed to be perfectly content as he munched along on a candy bar. In fact, that's what they called him— the "Candy Bar Man."

What the fans didn't know was that Casper was really a man in agony, trying to act normal. He suffered terrible headaches, muscle spasms, and sinus attacks. His greatest desire was to go to bed; drowsiness would beset him at the most inopportune times. The worse he felt, the more he turned to candy bars for comfort. The more he turned to candy bars, the more obese he became. The more obese he became —tipping the scale at 225 pounds at age thirty-two—the more exhausted he felt. There was scarcely a day he felt good.

Fortunately, his wife, in talking with a friend, heard about Dr. Randolph and cajoled her husband into going to see him. What he learned about himself in clinical testings came as a great shock and wiped out his usual breakfasts completely: he was allergic to eggs, citrus, and wheat. He was allergic to most of his other customary foods as well. That was in 1964.

Eventually, he was eating breakfasts of things like fried shrimp or swordfish, lunches of avocado or sardines, and dinners of elk stew or bear steak. But more than his diet had changed. So had his disposition and his waistline. And in 1965 he won the Vardon Trophy, professional golf's award for consistency—showing the benefits of a proper diet.

To understand the effectiveness of this diet, it is important to learn how it was determined what foods he could eat. The process began with a fasting period.

Fasting

The most effective way of determining food or chemical sensitivity is a process called comprehensive environmental control, developed by Dr. Randolph. Patients are diagnosed and treated in an ecology unit. The unit, usually one wing of a hospital, is cleared of all possible toxic substances (in the manner described later in the book as recommendations for nontoxic living). Patients are placed on a fast, being allowed only pure water, usually for four to seven days, until all allergic symptoms disappear. Then they are reexposed to foods and toxic substances one at a time, with enough of an interval to determine what is causing the allergic reaction.

We hope the day will soon come when every general hospital has such a unit, but as yet there is such a scarcity of ecologic units that some doctors have to let their patients go through the fasting period at home. Even though it is still done under the doctor's supervision, the picture which evolves of the patient's allergies is not so clear, since the patient could be reacting to things in the environment rather than to the foods being reintroduced into the diet.

We do not recommend that you try a do-it-yourself fast; you could become ill. Any fasting should be done under medical supervision. What you *can* do, if you want to test yourself, is use the rotary diversified diet, as described in this chapter, and keep a diary of foods eaten and symptoms experienced.

Although food is one of the greatest sources of nourishment, it is also one of the greatest stresses of life. Even at best, food puts a stress on the digestive system. So it follows that the greater the quantity of different foods, the greater the stress will be. Therefore, it is healthier to eat one food at a time.

Food Addiction

It can take up to four days to clear the food from the body including the gastrointestinal tract and other parts of the food absorption system. If you eat a particular food too frequently your system is never free from that food and you can become addicted to it in the same way that one becomes addicted to drugs. The treachery of food addiction is that you can become a food addict and not know it. The reason for that is the problem known as masking.

Masking

Let's assume you are allergic to peanuts. If for a period of ten days you avoid peanuts and everything made with them, you will probably have a very definite reaction shortly after reintroducing them into your diet. Delayed reaction can occur up to eighteen hours after eating.

If you keep on eating peanuts every day, you will have continuing reactions to a lesser degree. Soon you may not notice any reaction at all. This does not mean that you are no longer bothered by peanuts. The symptoms have merely been masked—hidden so they are no longer associated with the food that caused them. Other symptoms may appear; chronic ailments may develop. Eventually you may find that the only time you feel relief from certain complaints is after you have eaten peanuts. You begin to eat peanuts more and more often. When the problem reaches an acute state, you begin to crave them.

The cycle involved is very similar to drug addiction, with two additional problems that make the offender even more difficult to pinpoint. First, peanut oil is used in preparing many foods, so you are not always aware when peanuts are introduced into your system. Second, and even more confusing, is the fact that you may be addicted, in varying degrees, to several foods at once. The picture becomes so muddled that only an experienced clinician can solve the riddle.

Food addiction has been linked so often to schizophrenia, alcoholism, obesity, arthritis, and other disturbances, that we wonder why it is not common practice to pursue the rotary diversified diet as the first step in the treatment of these and other ailments.

Rotary Diversified Diet

The rotary diversified diet was devised by the late Dr. Herbert J. Rinkel, and those who have been helped to lead a normal life because of it are greatly indebted to him.

What is the rotary diet? It is an approach to eating that can prevent food allergies and addictions. It is a diet that can be used as a technique for uncovering and diagnosing food allergies and addictions. And finally it is a diet one can use for a short time or for the rest of one's life to treat food allergies and addictions.

Here is how it works. Only one food is eaten at a particular meal. You do not eat that food again until it has been cleared from your body —until at least four days later; this is usually a long enough interval.

Dr. Joseph Morgan maintains that, ideally, the best time to begin a rotary diversified diet is in infancy. If infants were fed this type of diet, the great majority of food allergies could be prevented. By teaching the child to eat one food at a time, he would never learn the bad eating habits which lead to addictions.

At the end of this chapter are four master plans showing four-day rotary diets. You can choose the one that suits you best. Or you can use it as a guide for making your own. As you learn to recognize food families, you will be able to vary your diet with food combinations to your taste. Also in this chapter you will find samples of diets for testing and/or management.

Prevention of Allergies

Even if your primary interest is just to modify your eating habits to prevent food allergies, it is recommended that you study this entire chapter on the rotary diversified diet and the introduction to Chapter 9 about food families. With an understanding of the principles of diagnosis and treatment, you'll be in a better position to decide the degree of prevention you wish to practice. For suggestions geared specifically to prevention, see "How to Change Your Eating Habits," p. 86.

A word of caution. With any severe illness—especially a heart condition—any history of mental illness, or any chronic unresolved medical complaints, do not consider using this diet for prevention; you may experience withdrawal symptoms which need to be treated immediately. You should attempt the rotary diversified diet only under the supervision of a physician who understands the problems involved.

MANAGEMENT OF COMPLEX FOOD ALLERGIES

Although a four-day rotation is recommended for prevention of food allergies, for treatment it is better that a food-allergic patient rotate foods in the diet at seven-day intervals, eating a different food for each of the twenty-one meals taken during the week. Some patients may be able to have a single-food snack in the evening, which constitutes a fourth feeding.

Let's take an example. The diet could begin on a Monday morning, day 1, with apples. No other food may be eaten with the apples for breakfast, but the patient can eat as many apples as desired. (For testing purposes only, there is a time limit of twenty minutes per meal.) Then apples will not be eaten again in any form until the following Monday morning, which begins the second rotation of the diet.

For lunch on Monday, he or she can eat sweet potatoes—and only sweet potatoes—steamed or baked, and seasoned only with sea salt. (Initially sea salt is the only seasoning that can be added to the foods; it can be used as frequently as desired.) Sweet potatoes would then not be eaten again until lunch on the following Monday.

Each subsequent week would be a duplication of the first week. This method of rotation preserves an individual's tolerance for non-offending foods (new food allergies can occur if the patient is overexposed to any given food).

An Optimistic Note

Before we delve into the mechanics of the seven-day rotary diet or the shorter versions, be assured that you may eventually be able to tolerate many more foods than you do initially. When you have been fasting, or when you have abruptly switched to a rotary diet, your system has unusually heightened sensitivity as a result, and mild food offenders may cause a stronger reaction than they normally would. But foods that cause only mild symptoms may be returned to the diet and be tolerated with little or no difficulty within a few weeks.

There also are cyclic or non-fixed allergies. These are the food allergies that come and go and may return again, depending on the frequency of exposure. They may vary in intensity, sometimes causing mild reactions, sometimes severe.

Actually, these non-fixed allergies constitute at least 50 percent and as much as 70 or 80 percent of a patient's food allergies. But by proper management on a rotary diet, even some of the foods which cause moderate to severe symptoms can eventually be eaten safely. The reason is that the body has had an appropriate rest period during which time tolerance to many offenders has been regained.

Not infrequently, some foods can be eaten without problems after only three to four weeks of abstinence, whereas another offending food cannot be returned to the diet until two, three, or even six months have elapsed. A few foods may be permanent or fixed allergens.

PLANNING YOUR ROTARY DIET FOR COMPLEX FOOD ALLERGIES

There is no such thing as a typical rotary diet since it is highly unlikely you can find two highly food-sensitive people with identical lists of dietary offenders. You must plan your diet to fit your particular problem.

Forget the stereotype meals. The highly allergic individual will have to modify his customary ways of eating and revise his ideas of what constitutes a breakfast. For example, the patient who tolerates none of the foods ordinarily associated with breakfast may find himself eating meat, poultry, fish, or vegetables for breakfast.

In the beginning, you should not be unduly concerned about a balanced diet. The priority is the elimination of foods which cause trouble. You must concentrate your efforts on regaining your health and not worry about supplementing your diet with vitamins and minerals. Many patients have maintained excellent health on rotary diets for years, during which time they could not tolerate such supplements. This does not negate the value of vitamins and minerals, it merely defines a basic priority—survival!

First you must master the rotary technique of dieting—preferably with a seven-day diet, but if that is not possible, a six-, five-, or even a four-day diet—using foods that do not cause troublesome reactions. After this method of eating has been learned, you can concentrate on adding new foods, planning meals consisting of several foods, and balancing the diet.

In planning your diet, it is important to know the availability of foods. If chemical sensitivities have been diagnosed, it is necessary to find sources of food and water that are relatively free from contaminants—preservatives, herbicides and pesticides—and additives. These foods are labeled as natural or organic. If you have been tested positive to chlorine, fluoride, or plastic, your water should be pure well water or spring water that is bottled in glass. Not all well water is pure.

Food Families

Now, about food. This book contains a whole section on food families. But for our present purposes, before selecting foods for a rotary diet, it is necessary to understand that foods are grouped in families and that related foods should be eaten at proper intervals.

If you are allergic to one member of a food family, you may react to other foods in the same plant family—fruits, vegetables, nuts, seeds— or in the same animal family—meat, fish, fowl.

In the vegetable category, for example, if you are severely affected by tomatoes, you may have a reaction to other members of the same family such as eggplant, potatoes, green peppers, or paprika. For best results, you should separate members of the same family by at least three days. If potatoes are eaten for breakfast Monday morning, you should wait at least until Thursday before eating another member of that family, such as green peppers. An easy way to remember this: Separate individual foods by seven days and members of food families by at least three days. (The three-day interval for related foods obviously applies only to the seven-day and not to the four-day rotation plan.)

Rotating Plant Samples. Let's take a look at how you can rotate members of the plant families:

Apples (Mon.); 4 days later (Fri.), pears (of the same family); 3 days later (Mon.), apples are repeated on the next rotation.

Squash (Tues.); 3 days later (Fri.), cantaloupe (of the same family); 4 days later (Tues.), squash is repeated on the next rotation.

Carrots (Wed.); 4 days later (Sun.), celery (of the same family); 3 days later (Wed.), carrots are repeated on the next rotation.

Some food-allergy patients find they have no trouble with meats, fish, and poultry as long as each individual food is rotated every four days. Other patients need to be even more careful regarding rotation of foods in these groups. But there's no lack of variety. In the next chapter, on food families, you'll find that the animal classifications include mollusks, crustaceans, fish, amphibians, reptiles, birds, and mammals.

Rotating Animal Samples. Now let's see how you can rotate members of animal families:

Monday, lamb (Bovine Family); 4 days later (Fri.), pork (Swine Family); 3 days later (Mon.), lamb is eaten on the next rotation.

Tuesday, salmon (Salmon Family); 4 days later (Sat.), sole, flounder, or halibut (Flounder Family); 3 days later (Tues.), salmon is eaten on the next rotation.

Wednesday, duck (Duck Family); 4 days later (Sun.), turkey (Turkey Family); 3 days later (Wed.), duck is repeated on the next rotation.

The following four diets can be used as samples for testing or management of allergies. If you are using Diet Plan 1 for testing and you have some reaction after eating apples for breakfast Monday morning, it could be a sign that you are sensitive to apples. However, you could also be reacting to a food you had eaten prior to this diet. The following Monday, if you again have the same reaction to apples, it is very likely you are allergic to apples. If you are not sure, the third time around should clarify it.

Sometimes it is necessary to follow the identical diet for three or more weeks to get a clear picture of which foods are bothering you. The picture is sometimes muddled by exposure to an excitant other than food. Also, it is possible that you are having delayed reactions—reacting as much as eighteen hours after a food is ingested—so you don't know which food is causing the problem. That is why we strongly recommend that you do this under the supervision of a knowledgeable doctor.

DIET PLAN 1

This is a sample of a diet avoiding beef, milk, all grains, chicken, eggs, tomatoes, and lettuce.

	Breakfast	**Lunch**	**Dinner**
Mon.	apples	squash	lamb or goat (Bovine Family)
Tues.	oranges	lima beans	salmon or trout (Salmon Family)
Wed.	apricots	carrots	duck or goose (Duck Family)
Thurs.	cantaloupe	sweet potatoes	lobster or shrimp (Crustaceans)
Fri.	pears	cabbage	pork (Swine Family)
Sat.	strawberries	peas	sole, flounder, or halibut (Flounder Family)
Sun.	bananas	celery	turkey (Turkey Family)

Variations in the selection of foods and the time of their ingestion can be made according to your tolerance and taste. You may prefer meat, fish, or poultry for breakfast or lunch instead of for dinner.

On Monday, any type of squash could be eaten, or you could have pumpkin. For Tuesday, instead of lima beans, you could substitute peanuts, soybeans, or any other peas or beans (all members of the same family). This does not necessarily mean that foods in the same family are interchangeable with each other; this is a possibility, but it must be established for you. Until it is established, you assume that if you select lima beans, you repeat lima beans every Tuesday for lunch. If you select soybeans, you repeat soy beans every Tuesday for lunch, etc.

You may prefer to use the foods higher in carbohydrate content (more filling) on days when lobster or fish is eaten, leaving foods with a smaller amount of carbohydrate to be eaten on days that meat is taken (which seems to be more filling). For example, sweet potatoes and lobster on the same day; cabbage and pork on the same day.

While millet is not a grain, it is in the same family and should be rotated in the diet as such.

According to your taste, instead of turkey or duck, you could substitute squab (Dove Family) or guinea fowl (Guinea Fowl Family), but not pheasant (Pheasant Family) which is in the same family as chicken.

DIET PLAN 2

This is the sample of a diet avoiding pork, chicken, eggs, lobster, wheat, peanuts, peas, beans, apples, and oranges.

	Breakfast	**Lunch**	**Dinner**
Mon.	cherries or nectarines	potatoes	beef (Bovine Family)
Tues.	oatmeal	lettuce	cod or haddock (Cod Family)
Wed.	bananas	cabbage	turkey (Turkey Family)
Thurs.	grapes	almonds	lamb (Bovine Family)
Fri.	rice	green peppers	crab or shrimp (Crustaceans)
Sat.	peaches or plums (prunes)	squash	halibut or sole (Flounder Family)
Sun.	blueberries	cashew nuts	duck or goose (Duck Family)

DIET PLAN 3

You may be one of an increasing number of very sensitive people who find they can eat very few fruits and vegetables even if they are organically grown. Your diet consists primarily of animal proteins. Diet 3 suggests some comparatively unfamiliar vegetables and fruits. Because so many kinds of animal protein are used, you will have to choose from a wider classification of animals.

	Breakfast	**Lunch**	**Dinner**
Mon.	beef	avocadoes	salmon (Salmon Family)
Tues.	lobster	Jerusalem artichokes	turkey (Turkey Family)
Wed.	millet	mangoes	rabbit (Hare Family)
Thurs.	frog's legs or bear	ñame	lamb (Bovine Family)
Fri.	tuna	malanga	pheasant (Pheasant Family)
Sat.	crab, llama, or antelope	yuca	moose, elk, reindeer (Deer Family)
Sun.	bay scallops, clams, or oysters	plantains	halibut or sole (Flounder Family)

This diet introduces some of the more exotic foods such as wild game and ñame and yuca, which are tubular vegetables from South America. For source, see "Unusual Foods" following Diet Plan 4, page 84.

DIET PLAN 4

This diet is designed for those people who find they can eat no grains and very few of the usual animal proteins and must depend on wild game and nuts.

	Breakfast	Lunch	Dinner
Mon.	cashew or pistachio nuts	pears	moose or buffalo (Deer Family)
Tues.	almonds	cantaloupe	rabbit (Hare Family)
Wed.	sunflower seeds or buckwheat	okra	goat (Bovine Family)
Thurs.	peanuts	ñame or avocado	reindeer or elk (Deer Family)
Fri.	coconut	cherries	guinea hen, pheasant, or squab (Pheasant Family)
Sat.	macadamia nuts	squash	antelope or llama (Pronghorn Family)
Sun.	pecans or walnuts	celery	frogs legs (Frog Family), squid (Mollusks) or turtle (Turtle Family)

Unusual Foods. Some people have become so food-sensitive that they can tolerate very few of the foods they previously ate. These people have learned to enjoy exotic foods, foods from other lands, and foods known usually only to the gourmet. A good source for exotic meats is Czimer Brothers, R.R. 1, Box 285, Lockport, Ill. 60441, tel: (815) 838-3503. They ship foods packed in dry ice to people all over the country. After trying buffalo, elk, reindeer, and moose, many people have learned to enjoy hippopotamus meat, elephant meat, whale, and bear.

In stores catering to Latin Americans, you can buy tropical vegetables such as yuca, ñame, and malanga. Macadamia nuts, mangoes, and papayas are just a few of the delicacies that have been introduced to people with food sensitivities.

Mechanics for Testing

It is very important to keep a diary which lists each food eaten and the time and degree of any reactions that you experience.

Don't be too sure of your first results. The first cycle of a rotary diet cannot be considered conclusive because during the first three days it will not be possible to determine if any symptoms that appear at this time are due to the foods being eaten during this period. The symptoms may be delayed reactions, or they may be withdrawal symptoms to foods that were discontinued on switching to the rotary diet.

Unless there is a moderately severe reaction to any food, the second week should be an exact duplication of the first. After following the diet for the second time, foods that provoked reactions on both occasions should be removed and not reintroduced for several months— and not until you have found a satisfactory diet with which you enjoy good health. Only then are you ready to retest offending foods.

If as foods are eliminated you find you do not have enough foods to stay on a seven-day diet, you may have to change to a six-day, a five-day, or even, if absolutely necessary, a four-day diet, which uses only a total of twelve foods. A few extremely food-sensitive patients have had to restrict themselves to eight foods, allowing only two meals a day for a cycle of four days.

If the reaction to a food is not conclusive and there are only vague symptoms, it may help to change the order of the foods, putting the suspected food on another day to ascertain if there is a problem of confusion caused by a delayed reaction to another food. Sometimes you may really be reacting to an excitant in the environment and not to a given food.

If you have a reaction to a food, you should not eat the next scheduled meal because this might cause additional symptoms and lead to further confusion regarding the overall situation. You must clear the digestive tract as quickly as possible and be free of any symptoms before eating the next food. (See page 181 for treatment of food reactions.)

Adding Foods. When the diet has been stabilized at the level of twenty-one foods for at least three or four cycles, you can begin adding other foods. You can also test cold pressed oils, rotating them so that you are using a different oil each time. You should test no more than one "new" food a day. Some clinical ecologists recommend that the testing be done in the morning, after a night's fast, before anything else is eaten; other physicians recommend that the new food be taken at the noon meal because they do not trust morning symptoms. Experiment to find which time of the day gives you the clearest picture.

It is good to retest foods, beginning first with those which caused mild symptoms and gradually adding those foods which caused progressively more severe reactions. If a food retested after one or two months continues to produce symptoms, you should wait another three months before testing it again. If unsuccessful, it should be retested after a further six months' abstinence.

If the symptoms recur, the food must be considered a fixed allergen. However, to make sure, you can wait for one or two years and retry the food. If it still causes symptoms there is very little likelihood that this food can ever be returned to the diet without some problems.

Prevention: How to Change Your Eating Habits

Some persons are so sick that they are forced to make drastic changes in their eating habits; others do so out of choice. This section is addressed specifically to those of you who are health-oriented or mildly allergic. Most of you will fit into a category somewhere between the two extremes.

Begin by simplifying your diet. Learn to savor the flavor of individual foods; you'll find them much more enjoyable than when they are masked with sauces and gravies.

We have collected ideas from many people who have told us how they made the transition to a healthier diet. Here are some suggestions for those who prefer gradual changes.

1. Accept the fact that there will be times when you have little choice in foods, as when traveling or eating out. However, don't use that as an excuse to continue an unhealthy diet. You can usually find a good compromise.

2. Keep track of the foods you eat. Vary your foods. If you are following the rotary diet for allergy prevention, it is not necessary to concern yourself with separating individual foods by more than four days.

The diets suggested earlier in the chapter are designed to reveal a pattern of allergic reaction and that is why the foods *must* be repeated in the same pattern week after week without exception until your reaction to each food is fully understood. After it has been established, however, you can use your discretion on how often to eat any given food. Those foods which you particularly like you can repeat, leaving only a four-day interval. For variety's sake, you can rotate all the other foods at any longer interval.

3. Avoid prepackaged foods; accept the fact that there is no way for you to know all their ingredients. When the label says the product contains vegetable oil, it could be a blend of vegetable oils including soy oil, peanut oil, corn oil, etc. Most canned and frozen foods have some form of corn in them. That is one of the reasons why so many people in the United States are addicted to corn.

4. Choose only natural foods without additives—no preservatives, no artificial coloring, no artificial flavors.

5. Whenever possible, buy foods grown without chemical fertilizers or pesticides. If you are fortunate enough to have your own garden, make sure that you grow your vegetables organically.

6. Begin to eliminate sugar, white flour, and white rice from your diet. Do not substitute raw sugar. Raw sugar is filled with bacteria. Besides, sugar in any form is a stress food; substitute whole-wheat flour for white flour and brown rice for white rice.

7. In the beginning, you may prefer eating multiple-food meals, because you are accustomed to them. Try to plan them so you are eating no more than three or four food families at a time.

You will recall that Billy Casper ate such things as swordfish for breakfast and elk stew for dinner. He preferred multiple-food meals and ate tomatoes with his swordfish and eggplant with his elk. For the most part, the recipes in this book are limited to three or four food families.

8. Select a food that you thoroughly enjoy—a fruit, a vegetable, or any protein such as meat, fish, eggs; eat nothing but that food at one meal, but eat as much as you desire.

You may decide to eat six or eight eggs. The quantity may surprise you, but since you won't be eating eggs again for at least another four days, that is permissible. Salt to taste.

Find as many single-food meals as you can. Gradually you'll build up a taste for a one-food meal. Fruits and raw vegetables are especially suitable; they're the easiest kind of meal that you can take to work for lunch. You'll have to experiment to find how large a portion you need. One woman eats eight bananas at a meal, while another is satisfied with just four. Four or five apples satisfy most people.

If you're having corn as your one-dish meal, steam the corn, then season it with cold pressed corn oil and salt. One patient found she could eat one or two large bowls of popcorn once a week without adding to her weight. Before going on her rotary diet, she says, she gained weight just by looking at corn. Try different combinations and you will be surprised at how many new meals you will enjoy. One woman who did not like squash learned that if she combined zucchini and yellow summer squash, steamed it, salted it, and added two tablespoons of oil, she found it a very tasty dish. If she used almond oil she could eat almonds with it.

Keep your meals as simple as possible. If you are eating organic foods for the first time, it will come as a big surprise how delicious fruits and vegetables are. It did not take us long to discover that chemicals and additives camouflage the natural sweetness of foods.

We were amazed to find that we no longer needed sugar or honey to sweeten grapefruit and cantaloupe (which we used to douse with sugar). People who once craved candy and ice cream report that a beautiful organic persimmon or a tasty nectarine is more satisfying than the sweets they used to crave but which were so stressful to them.

Weight Control

Would you believe that the same type of diet helps overweight people lose weight and underweight people gain weight? This is no gimmick. It is a scientifically proven fact and easily explained.

To give just one illustration of how the rotary diversified diet helps you gain weight, consider the problem of diarrhea. Diarrhea is frequently a symptom of food allergy. By rotating your foods you learn to avoid those foods that cause diarrhea—and naturally you begin to gain weight.

On the other hand, by going on a rotary diversified diet, one woman was able to lose fifty pounds though she was eating more than she had with other diets that made her gain weight. This merely proves it is not necessarily how much you eat, but what you eat, and even more important, how frequently you eat it.

Naturally, if you don't break away from the foods to which you are addicted, you will continue to crave them and never feel satisfied. You'll always be eating—and, of course, gaining weight. Another major contributor to weight gain is *napping right after you eat*. And since two of the most frequent symptoms of food allergies are drowsiness and hunger, is it any wonder that clinical ecologists are convinced that the safest, the healthiest, and the most pleasurable way of losing weight is by following the rotary diversified diet? Pleasurable? Of course! Once you've stabilized your diet you're never hungry; you're always satisfied.

Other Benefits

So many people who pursue rotary diversified diets report that they really feel much better than they ever felt in their lives. After they discovered their food allergies, a lot of backaches and headaches and other minor ailments that they assumed were just a part of living were cleared up as a result of going on this diet.

One man, who had been injured while playing basketball in high school, assumed that the backaches he had had all his adult years were a result of that injury. He did not know what it was to wake up without a backache. He was quite surprised to find that after he began following a rotary diversified diet, the backaches disappeared.

But more important even than the freedom from pain is a newfound energy. People have reported that all their lives they had felt sluggish and fatigued, dragging their feet; then suddenly, after stabilizing their rotary diversified diet, they were brimming with energy. Men and women in their forties and fifties find that they have, in spite of serious allergies, more energy and stamina than young people in their twenties. One woman said that the greatest bonus she receives when she conscientiously follows her rotary diversified diet is that she looks and feels and acts ten years younger.

Is that an incentive to you? It is to many people.

How to Choose Your Diet

Until you have learned all the techniques of the rotary diversified diet and can select other foods and food combinations in accordance with your taste, the four diet charts below can serve as guidelines. Notice that all four charts suggest meat for the first day, fish for the second day, fowl and eggs for the third, and shellfish for the fourth. The diets also show how you can vary vegetables, fruits, oils, etc., to go with your day's food.

For the mildly allergic who may have an allergy to only one thing, the charts must be modified for individual needs. For example, for someone sensitive to all shellfish, you would have to substitute with a fish family not used on your fish day.

Select one of the charts according to your taste. For example, you may prefer Chart 1, because your chicken and onion meals are on the same day. Or you may prefer Chart 4, which has potatoes and tomatoes with your chicken. These food combinations were not chosen lightly. The foods belong to certain families. As long as you use only the foods listed for day 1 and do not repeat them until the fifth day, you will be following a proper four-day rotation.

If you look at Chart 1, you will see how much of a variety you have. For example, on day 1 you can have squash, pumpkin, or cucumber as your vegetable and at the same meal have any melon or cantaloupe for dessert. No member of that family will appear on day 2, 3, or 4. If you are having one of those vegetables for lunch but would like to have another vegetable for dinner, you still have a selection. Since you should not eat squash or any other member of the Gourd Family twice on the same day, you can choose corn or yams, both of which are in a different family. Or if you chose corn or bamboo shoots as your vegetable, you can also eat other members of the grass family, the grains such as wheat, rye, and barley. Note that you have vinegar (a yeast), cheese (a mold), and mushrooms all on the same day. That is because they are all of the Fungi Family.

After you have gone through your four-day diet, it is not necessary for you to eat the precise foods you chose the first time around. You can choose a different food as long as you stay within the limits of that

CHART 1: SAMPLE ROTARY DIVERSIFIED DIET

	Day 1	Day 2	Day 3	Day 4
Protein	*All red meats and their products* Beef, veal, lamb, buffalo, goat. Pork. Venison. Milk, yogurt, all cheeses.	*All fish* Haddock, cod. Perch. Carp. Tuna, mackerel. Rock cod. Turbot, sole, halibut, flounder. Trout, salmon. Sardines, herring. Red snapper.	*Fowl and eggs* Chicken, pheasant, guinea hen. Turkey, goose, duck. Eggs.	*Shellfish* Clams, oysters. Crab, shrimp, lobster. Snails, squid. Scallops. Abalone.
Vegetables	Squash, zucchini, pumpkin, cucumber. Mushrooms. Corn, bamboo shoots. Yams.	Potatoes, tomatoes, eggplant, peppers. Lettuce, artichokes, dandelions, endive. Carrots, parsley, parsnips, celery. Yuca.	Spinach, beets, Swiss chard. Asparagus, onions, leeks. Okra. Sweet potatoes.	All peas and beans, lentils, soy, alfalfa sprouts, bean sprouts (legumes). Cabbage, broccoli, turnips, radishes, cauliflower, kohlrabi, rutabaga, Brussels sprouts, mustard greens, kale. Water chestnuts.
Fruit	Apples, pears. Strawberries, raspberries, blackberries, boysenberries. All melons. Mangoes. Guavas.	Oranges, grapefruit, lemons, tangerines, kumquats. Pineapple. Avocado. Currants, gooseberries. Rhubarb.	Peaches, apricots, nectarines, plums, prunes, cherries. Papayas. Persimmons. Dates.	Blueberries, cranberries, huckleberries. Grapes, raisins. Bananas. Pomegranates. Figs.

Seeds and Nuts	Cashews, pistachios. Filberts, hazelnuts. Pumpkin seeds.	Pecans, walnuts. Sunflower seeds.	Almonds. Brazil nuts. Macadamia nuts.	Peanuts, soy nuts. Sesame seeds. Pine nuts.
Other	Yeast, apple vinegar. Wheat, rye, barley, cane, corn meal, popcorn, millet, oats, rice. Olives. Gelatin.	Buckwheat. Tapioca. Sunflower meal.	Coconut. Arrowroot starch.	Peanut butter. Carob. Sesame meal.
Sweeteners	Molasses, malt syrup. Whey, lactose.	Maple sugar or syrup. Avocado honey.* Buckwheat honey.*	Date sugar. Sage honey.*	Clover honey.*
Fats and Oils	Corn oil, olive oil. Butter, lard, beef fat.	Safflower oil, sunflower oil. Walnut oil. Any fish oil.	Cottonseed oil. Coconut oil. Almond oil. Chicken fat, turkey fat.	Peanut oil. soy oil. Sesame oil.
Herbs and Spices	Vanilla bean. Black pepper. Allspice, cloves.	Chili, pimiento, paprika, cayenne, red pepper. Cinnamon, bay leaf. Dill, caraway, fennel, anise, chervil, cumin, coriander.	Garlic, chives. Mint, sage, marjoram, basil, rosemary, oregano, thyme. Ginger, cardamon, turmeric.	Mustard. Horseradish. Cream of tartar. Nutmeg, mace.
Teas	Comfrey. Rosehips. Sarsaparilla.	Chamomile, goldenrod. Parsley. Sassafras.	Papaya leaf. Mint.	Blueberry leaf. Alfalfa. Juniper berry. Hops. Senna.

*Honey can be used only once in four days.

CHART 2: SAMPLE ROTARY DIVERSIFIED DIET

	Day 1	Day 2	Day 3	Day 4
Protein	*All red meats and their products* Beef, veal, lamb, buffalo, goat. Pork. Venison. Milk, yogurt, all cheeses.	*All fish* Haddock, cod. Perch. Carp. Tuna, mackerel. Rock cod. Turbot, sole, halibut, flounder. Trout, salmon. Sardines, herring. Red snapper.	*Fowl and eggs* Chicken, pheasant, guinea hen. Turkey, goose, duck. Eggs.	*Shellfish* Clams, oysters. Crab, shrimp, lobster. Snails, squid. Scallops. Abalone.
Vegetables	Squash, zucchini, pumpkin, cucumber. Mushrooms. Sweet potatoes. Water chestnuts.	Lettuce, artichokes, dandelions, endive. Cabbage, broccoli, turnips, radishes, cauliflower, kohlrabi, rutabaga, Brussels sprouts, mustard greens, kale. Yams, yuca.	All peas and beans, lentils, soy, alfalfa sprouts, bean sprouts (legumes). Carrots, celery, parsnips, parsley. Asparagus, onions, leeks.	Potatoes, tomatoes, eggplant, peppers. Spinach, beets, Swiss chard. Okra. Corn, bamboo shoots.
Fruit	Peaches, apricots, nectarines, cherries, plums, prunes. All melons. Pineapple. Dates.	Bananas. Grapes, raisins. Blueberries, cranberries, huckleberries. Persimmons. Guavas.	Apples, pears. Strawberries, raspberries, blackberries, boysenberries. Papayas. Rhubarb. Mangoes. Currants.	Oranges, grapefruit, lemons, tangerines, kumquats. Avocado. Pomegranates. Figs. Gooseberries.

Seeds and Nuts	Almonds. Pumpkin seeds. Macadamia nuts.	Pecans, walnuts. Sunflower seeds.	Peanuts, soy nuts. Cashews, pistachios. Sesame seeds.	Brazil nuts. Filberts, hazelnuts, chestnuts. Pine nuts.
Other	Yeast. Coconut. Arrowroot starch. Gelatin.	Sunflower meal. Tapioca.	Buckwheat. Sesame meal. Peanut butter.	Wheat, rye, barley, cornmeal, popcorn, cane, oats, rice, millet. Olives.
Sweeteners	Date sugar. Whey, lactose.	Maple sugar or syrup. Sage honey.*	Clover honey.* Buckwheat honey.*	Avocado honey.* Molasses, malt syrup.
Fats and Oils	Butter, lard, beef fat. Almond oil. Coconut oil.	Safflower oil, sunflower oil. Walnut oil. Any fish oils.	Peanut oil, soy oil. Sesame oil. Chicken fat, turkey fat.	Corn oil. Cottonseed oil. Olive oil.
Herbs and Spices	Black pepper. Nutmeg, mace. Vanilla bean.	Mint, sage, rosemary, basil, marjoram, oregano, thyme. Mustard, horseradish. Cream of tartar. Allspice, cloves.	Garlic, chives. Ginger, cardamon, turmeric. Dill, fennel, caraway, anise, chervil, cumin, coriander.	Chili, pimiento, paprika, cayenne, red pepper. Cinnamon, bay leaf.
Teas	Rosehips.	Chamomile, goldenrod. Blueberry. Mint.	Parsley. Alfalfa. Papaya leaf. Senna. Sarsaparilla.	Juniper berry. Comfrey. Hops. Sassafras.

*Honey can be used only once in four days.

CHART 3: SAMPLE ROTARY DIVERSIFIED DIET

	Day 1	Day 2	Day 3	Day 4
Protein	*All red meats and their products* Beef, veal, lamb, buffalo, goat. Pork. Venison. Milk, yogurt, all cheeses.	*Shellfish* Clams, oysters. Crabs, shrimp, lobster. Snails, squid. Scallops. Abalone.	*Fowl and eggs* Chicken, pheasant, guinea hen. Turkey, duck, goose. Eggs.	*All fish* Haddock, cod. Perch. Carp. Tuna, mackerel. Rock cod. Turbot, sole, halibut, flounder. Trout, salmon. Sardines, herring. Red snapper.
Vegetables	Lettuce, artichokes, endive, dandelions. Potatoes, tomatoes, eggplant, peppers. Mushrooms. Yams.	All peas and beans, lentils, alfalfa sprouts, bean sprouts, soy (legumes). Spinach, beets, Swiss chard. Yuca.	Carrots, parsley, celery, parsnips. Squash, zucchini, pumpkin, cucumber. Okra.	Cabbage, broccoli, turnips, radishes, cauliflower, kale, kohlrabi, rutabaga, Brussels sprouts, mustard greens. Sweet potatoes. Asparagus, onions, leeks. Corn, bamboo shoots.
Fruit	Apples, pears. Strawberries, raspberries, blackberries, boysenberries. Papayas. Figs.	Peaches, apricots, nectarines, cherries, plums, prunes. Pineapple. Persimmons. Currants. Gooseberries.	All melons. Avocado. Rhubarb. Bananas. Dates. Mangoes.	Oranges, grapefruit, lemons, tangerines, kumquats. Blueberries, cranberries, huckleberries. Grapes, raisins. Pomegranates. Guavas.

Seeds and Nuts	Pecans, walnuts. Sesame seeds. Macadamia nuts.	Brazil nuts. Cashews, pistachio nuts. Pumpkin seeds.	Peanuts, soy nuts. Almonds.	Sunflower seeds. Filberts, hazelnuts, chestnuts. Pine nuts.
Other	Wheat, rye, barley, cornmeal, popcorn, cane, rice, oats, millet. Sesame meal.	Olives. Buckwheat. Coconut.	Peanut butter. Carob. Tapioca.	Yeast, apple vinegar. Sunflower meal. Arrowroot. Gelatin.
Sweeteners	Molasses, malt syrup.	Date sugar. Avocado honey.* Buckwheat honey.*	Clover honey.* Sage honey.*	Whey, lactose. Maple sugar or syrup.
Fats and Oils	Corn oil, sesame oil. Walnut oil. Any fish oil.	Cottonseed oil. Coconut oil. Olive oil. Chicken fat, turkey fat.	Peanut oil, soy oil. Almond oil.	Safflower oil, sunflower oil. Butter, lard, beef fat.
Herbs and Spices	Mustard, horseradish. Cream of tartar. Garlic, chives. Allspice, cloves.	Dill, caraway, fennel, cumin, anise, chervil, coriander. Cinnamon, bay leaf.	Mint, sage, rosemary, basil, oregano, marjoram, thyme. Ginger, cardamon, turmeric. Vanilla bean.	Chili, paprika, pimiento, cayenne, red pepper. Nutmeg, mace.
Teas	Blueberry leaf. Sarsaparilla.	Parsley. Sassafras. Comfrey.	Rosehips. Alfalfa. Mint. Senna.	Chamomile, goldenrod. Papaya leaf. Hops. Juniper berry.

*Honey can be used only once in four days.

CHART 4: SAMPLE ROTARY DIVERSIFIED DIET

	Day 1	Day 2	Day 3	Day 4
Protein	*All red meats and their products* Beef, veal, lamb, buffalo, goat. Pork. Venison. Milk, yogurt, all cheeses.	*Shellfish* Clams, oysters. Crab, shrimp, lobster. Snails. Squid. Scallops.	*Fowl and eggs* Chicken, pheasant, guinea hen. Turkey, goose, duck. Eggs.	*All fish* Haddock, cod. Perch. Carp. Tuna, mackerel. Rock cod. Turbot, sole, halibut, flounder. Trout, salmon. Sardines, herring. Red snapper.
Vegetables	Mushrooms. Cabbage, broccoli, turnips, kale, radishes, cauliflower, kohlrabi, rutabaga, Brussels sprouts, mustard greens. Asparagus, onions, leeks, yuca. Yams.	Lettuce, artichokes, endive, dandelions. Carrots, celery, parsnips, parsley. Sweet potatoes.	Potatoes, eggplant, tomatoes, peppers. Spinach, beets, Swiss chard. Corn, bamboo shoots.	All peas and beans, lentils, alfalfa sprouts, bean sprouts, soy (legumes). Okra. Squash, pumpkin, zucchini, cucumber.
Fruits	Bananas. Avocado. Pineapple. Pomegranates. Currants. Gooseberries.	Peaches, apricots, nectarines, cherries, plums, prunes. Apples, pears. Strawberries, raspberries, blackberries, boysenberries. Guavas.	Oranges, grapefruit, lemons, tangerines, kumquats. Grapes, raisins. Persimmons. Mangoes. Dates. Coconut.	All melons. Blueberries, cranberries, huckleberries. Papayas. Figs. Rhubarb.

Seeds and Nuts	Pecans, walnuts. Sesame seeds. Pine nuts.	Sunflower seeds. Almonds.	Brazil nuts. Cashews, pistachios. Macadamia nuts.	Peanuts, soy nuts. Pumpkin seeds. Filberts, hazelnuts, chestnuts.
Other	Yeast. Sesame meal. Tapioca. Gelatin.	Sunflower meal. Arrowroot starch.	Wheat, rye, barley, cornmeal, popcorn, cane, oats, rice, millet. Olives.	Buckwheat.
Sweeteners	Whey, lactose. Avocado honey.*	Maple sugar or syrup.	Date sugar. Molasses, malt syrup.	Clover honey.* Buckwheat honey.* Sage honey.*
Fats and Oils	Butter, lard, beef fat. Sesame oil. Walnut oil.	Sunflower oil, safflower oil. Almond oil.	Corn oil. Coconut oil. Olive oil. Chicken fat, turkey fat.	Peanut oil, soy oil. Any fish oil.
Herbs and Spices	Cinnamon, bay leaf. Mustard, horseradish. Vanilla bean. Garlic, chives.	Dill, fennel, caraway, anise, chervil, cumin, coriander. Allspice, cloves.	Cream of tartar. Chili, pimiento, paprika, cayenne, red pepper. Ginger, cardamon, turmeric.	Mint, sage, marjoram, basil, rosemary, oregano, thyme. Nutmeg, mace.
Teas	Sassafras. Juniper berry.	Chamomile, goldenrod. Parsley. Rosehips.	Comfrey.	Mint. Hops. Senna. Blueberry leaf. Alfalfa. Papaya leaf.

*Honey can be used only once in four days.

day. In other words, if you ate raspberries the first time around on day 1, you may decide to eat cantaloupe or mango the second time around.

Honey contains bee protein and can be used only once in four days regardless of its source. Therefore, if you are using avocado honey on day 2, you cannot use sage honey on day 3, even though they come from different families.

Select the chart that you would like to try first and post it in your kitchen. It is not advisable to use more than three foods at any one meal. Keep in mind that this suggestion is for the middle-of-the-road people, those who are using these charts for allergy prevention or to maintain good health. We still believe that the ideal method of eating is one food for each meal—three or four foods a day. And many persons with complex allergies do just that even after their allergies are under control.

CHAPTER 9

Introduction to Food Families

DEPRIVED OF things to eat? Far from it. We are going to introduce you to a whole new world of foods.

Man has restricted himself in the plants and animals around which he has built his diet. As a result, he eats only a small percentage of the edible foods of the world. Treat the fact that you are allergic to some foods as a challenge to devise a more exciting diet. Use the lists that follow to explore a variety of possibilities, adding new foods like yuca, malanga, kiwi, and comfrey to your diet.

You will notice that the lists include more than just foods. They include plants that you can smell, rub on yourself, and enjoy in many ways. Use the food families to find new beverages and new herbs. You may even decide to grow your own herbs and plants. *Be adventurous!*

How to Use the Numbers. There is a number in front of each item in the alphabetical listing of foods and related products (List 1, page 100). If you want to know other foods or products of the same family, turn to that number in the list of food families (List 2, page 108). In other words, List 1 is an alphabetical list of foods and related products and List 2 is a corresponding numerical list we have devised to make it easier for you to find your way through the food families.

Let's say you are allergic to cucumbers. You now need to know whether there are other members of the same family that may cause you trouble. In front of "cucumber" in List 1 is the number 79. You check 79 in List 2 and find that there is a long list of foods to which it is quite likely you are also allergic—pumpkins, squash, and cantaloupe, to mention just a few—all members of the Gourd Family. When you are planning your rotary diversified diet, you must allow for the fact that the Rose Family differs from the others in that for some unknown reason the four subdivisions—pomes, stone fruits, berries, and herbs—can usually be treated as if they were different families. If necessary, pomes (apples and pears) can be eaten on Monday; stone fruits (almonds, peaches, apricots) on Tuesday; berries (blackberries and raspberries) on Wednesday.

There are people so sensitive they are allergic to all four divisions,

99

but not as a general rule. Then there are those who are allergic to apples and who must be careful with pears (same subdivision), but not necessarily with peaches and cherries (a different subdivision).

Interestingly, not all berries are members of the Rose Family. Blueberries belong to the Heath Family, elderberries, to the Honeysuckle Family, gooseberries, to the Saxifrage Family, and these can be rotated accordingly.

Beverages. When using List 2, you'll notice there is an asterisk in front of certain foods. This means that one or more parts of the plant can be used in making beverages. (If you make beverages, be sure to coordinate the plant with your rotary diversified diet.)

Scientific Names. In addition to the recognizable names, the lists include scientific names of the food families. The purpose is to clarify certain discrepancies. For example, there are eight sources of arrowroot, only one of which is in the Arrowroot Family. Arrowroot (*Musa*) is in the Banana Family, and East Indian arrowroot (*Curcuma*) is in the Ginger Family. Arrowroot (*Maranta* starch) is in the Arrowroot Family. When buying arrowroot starch, if you cannot discover its source, you have to consider all eight families as one family in planning your rotary diversified diet.

Caution: Non-edible Plants. For a very good reason, you will find non-edible plants included in the lists. Some persons are highly sensitive to non-edible plants which are related to certain foods. For example, if you are allergic to poison ivy, you should probably avoid cashews, pistachios, and mangoes—see family 48.

Here is a comprehensive list of foods from *A* to *Z*—from abalone to zucchini—and the number of the family to which each belongs.[1] The individual foods are written in small letters, and the names of the food families are capitalized.

LIST 1
FOOD FAMILIES (ALPHABETICAL)

A

81	abalone	1	Algae
80	absinthe	63	allspice
41	acacia (gum)	40b	almond
46	acerola	11	*Aloe vera*
79	acorn squash	54	althea root
1	agar agar	12	Amaryllis Family
12	agave	94	amberjack
98	albacore	86	American eel
41	alfalfa	117	Amphibians

85	anchovy
65	angelica
65	anise
38	annatto
136	antelope
40a	apple
73	apple mint
40b	apricot
47	arrowroot, Brazilian (tapioca)
9	arrowroot (*Colocasia*)
17	arrowroot, East Indian (*Curcuma*)
19	Arrowroot Family
13	arrowroot, Fiji (*Tacca*)
4	arrowroot, Florida (*Zamia*)
19	arrowroot (*Maranta* starch)
16	arrowroot (*Musa*)
18	arrowroot, Queensland
80	artichoke flour
9	Arum Family
11	asparagus
2	*Aspergillus*
34	avocado

B

2	baker's yeast
6	bamboo shoots
16	banana
16	Banana Family
46	Barbados cherry
6	barley
73	basil
114	bass (black)
113	bass (yellow)
53	basswood
34	bay leaf
41	bean
132	bear
66	bearberry
24	Beech Family
137	beef
28	beet
74	bell pepper
73	bergamot
23	Birch Family
121	birds
38	Bixa Family

114	black bass
40c	blackberry
41	black-eyed peas
21	black pepper
80	black salsify
22	black walnut
66	blueberry
93	bluefish
80	boneset
98	bonito
79	Boston marrow
71	borage
71	Borage Family
40c	boysenberry
137	Bovine Family
6	bran
52	brandy
47	Brazilian arrowroot
62	Brazil nut
25	breadfruit
2	brewer's yeast
36	broccoli
36	Brussels sprouts
27	buckwheat
27	Buckwheat Family
6	bulgur
80	burdock root
40	burnet
31	Buttercup Family
79	buttercup squash
101	butterfish
22	butternut
79	butternut squash

C

36	cabbage
55	cacao
60	Cactus Family
6	cane sugar
18	Canna Family
79	cantaloupe
37	caper
37	Caper Family
74	*Capsicum*
42	carambola
65	caraway seed
17	cardamon

36   watercress
79   watermelon
96   weakfish
131 whale
61   wheat
61   wheat germ
90   whitebait
107 whitefish
21   white pepper
113 white perch
6   wild rice
40c wineberry
52   wine vinegar
23   wintergreen
73   winter savory
80   witloof chicory
76   woodruff
80   wormwood

Y

14   yam
14   Yam Family
14   yampi
80   yarrow
9   yautia
113 yellow bass
94   yellow jack
115 yellow perch
49   yerba maté
40c youngberry
47   yuca
11   yucca

Z

4   *Zamia*
79   zucchini

LIST 2
FOOD FAMILIES (NUMERICAL)

Plant

1 Algae
     agar agar
     carrageen (Irish moss)
     *dulse
     kelp (seaweed)
2 Fungi
     baker's yeast ("Red Star")
     brewer's or nutritional yeast
     mold (in certain cheeses)
         citric acid (*Aspergillus*)
     morel
     mushroom
     puffball
     truffle
3 Horsetail Family, *Equisetaceae*
     *shavegrass (horsetail)
4 Cycad Family, *Cycadaceae*
     Florida arrowroot (*Zamia*)
5 Conifer Family, *Coniferae*
     *juniper (gin)
     pine nut (piñon, pinyon)

6 Grass Family, *Gramineae*
     barley
       malt
       maltose
     bamboo shoots
     corn (mature)
       corn meal
       corn oil
       cornstarch
       corn sugar
       corn syrup
       hominy grits
       popcorn
     lemon grass
       citronella
     millet
     oat
       oatmeal
     rice
       rice flour
     rye

*One or more plant parts (leaf, root, seed, etc.) used as a beverage.

sorghum grain
  syrup
sugar cane
  cane sugar
  molasses
  raw sugar
sweet corn
triticale
wheat
  bran
  bulgur
  flour
    gluten
    graham
    patent
    whole wheat
  wheat germ
wild rice
7 Sedge Family, Cyperaceae
  Chinese water chestnut
  chufa (groundnut)
8 Palm Family, Palmaceae
  coconut
    coconut meal
    coconut oil
  date
    date sugar
  palm cabbage
  sago starch (Metroxylon)
9 Arum Family, Araceae
  ceriman (Monstera)
  dasheen (Colocasia)
    arrowroot
  taro (Colocasia) arrowroot
    poi
  malanga (Xanthosoma)
  yautia (Xanthosoma)
10 Pineapple Family, Bromeliaceae
  pineapple
11 Lily Family, Liliaceae
  Aloe vera
  asparagus
  chives
  garlic
  leek
  onion

ramp
*sarsaparilla
shallot
yucca (soap plant)
12 Amaryllis Family, Amaryllidaceae
  agave
    mescal, pulque, and tequila
13 Tacca Family, Taccaceae
  Fiji arrowroot (Tacca)
14 Yam Family, Dioscoreaceae
  Chinese potato (yam)
  ñame (yampi)
15 Iris Family, Iridaceae
  orris root (scent)
  saffron (Crocus)
16 Banana Family, Musaceae
  arrowroot (Musa)
  banana
  plantain
17 Ginger Family, Zingiberaceae
  cardamon
  East Indian arrowroot (Curcuma)
  ginger
  turmeric
18 Canna Family, Cannaceae
  Queensland arrowroot
19 Arrowroot Family, Marantaceae
  arrowroot (Maranta starch)
20 Orchid Family, Orchidaceae
  vanilla
21 Pepper Family, Piperaceae
  peppercorn (Piper)
    black pepper
    white pepper
22 Walnut Family, Juglandaceae
  black walnut
  butternut
  English walnut
  heartnut
  hickory nut
  pecan
23 Birch Family, Betulaceae
  filbert (hazelnut)
  oil of birch (wintergreen)

(some wintergreen flavor is methyl salicylate)

24 Beech Family, *Fagaceae*
    chestnut
    chinquapin
25 Mulberry Family, *Moraceae*
    breadfruit
    fig
    *hop
    mulberry
26 Protea Family, *Proteaceae*
    macadamia (Queensland nut)
27 Buckwheat Family,
            Polygonaceae
    buckwheat
    garden sorrel
    rhubarb
    sea grape
28 Goosefoot Family,
            Chenopodiaceae
    beet
    chard
    lamb's-quarters
    spinach
    sugar beet
    tampala
29 Carpetweed Family, *Aizoaceae*
    New Zealand spinach
30 Purslane Family, *Portulacaceae*
    pigweed (purslane)
31 Buttercup Family,
            Ranunculaceae
    *golden seal
32 Custard-Apple Family
    Annona species
    custard-apple
    papaw (pawpaw)
33 Nutmeg Family, *Myristicaceae*
    nutmeg
    mace
34 Laurel Family, *Lauraceae*
    avocado
    bay leaf
    cassia bark
    cinnamon
    *sassafras
        filé (powdered leaves)

35 Poppy Family, *Papaveraceae*
    poppyseed
36 Mustard Family, *Cruciferae*
    broccoli
    Brussels sprouts
    cabbage
    cardoon
    cauliflower
    Chinese cabbage
    collards
    colza shoots
    couve tronchuda
    curly cress
    horseradish
    kale
    kohlrabi
    mustard greens
    mustard seed
    radish
    rape
    rutabaga (swede)
    turnip
    upland cress
    watercress
37 Caper Family, *Capparidaceae*
    caper
38 Bixa Family, *Bixaceae*
    annatto (natural yellow dye)
39 Saxifrage Family,
            Saxifragaceae
    currant
    gooseberry
40 Rose Family, *Rosaceae*
    a. pomes
        apple
        cider
            vinegar
        pectin
        crabapple
        loquat
        pear
        quince
        *rosehips
    b. *stone fruits*
        almond
        apricot
        cherry

peach (nectarine)
plum (prune)
sloe
c. *berries*
  blackberry
  boysenberry
  dewberry
  loganberry
  longberry
  youngberry
  *raspberry (leaf)
  black raspberry
  red raspberry
  purple raspberry
  *strawberry (leaf)
  wineberry
d. *herb*
  burnet (cucumber flavor)

41   Legume Family, *Leguminoseae*
*alfalfa (sprouts)
beans
  fava
  lima
  mung (sprouts)
  navy
  string (kidney)
black-eyed pea (cowpea)
*carob
  carob syrup
chickpea (garbanzo)
*fenugreek
gum acacia
gum tragacanth
jicama
kudzu
lentil
*licorice
pea
peanut
  peanut oil
*red clover
*senna
soybean
  lecithin
  soy flour
  soy grits
  soy milk

soy oil
tamarind
tonka bean
  coumarin

42   Oxalis Family, *Oxalidaceae*
carambola
oxalis

43   Nasturtium Family,
       Tropaeolaceae
nasturtium

44   Flax Family, *Linaceae*
*flaxseed

45   Rue (Citrus) Family, *Rutaceae*
citron
grapefruit
kumquat
lemon
lime
murcot
orange
pummelo
tangelo
tangerine

46   Malpighia Family,
       Malpighiaceae
acerola (Barbados cherry)

47   Spurge Family, *Euphorbiaceae*
cassava or yuca (*Manihot*)
  cassava meal
  tapioca (Brazilian
    arrowroot)
castor bean
  castor oil

48   Cashew Family, *Anacardiaceae*
cashew
mango
pistachio
poison ivy
poison oak
poison sumac

49   Holly Family, *Aquifoliaceae*
maté (yerba maté)

50   Maple Family
maple sugar
maple syrup

51   Soapberry Family, *Sapindaceae*
litchi (lychee)

52 Grape Family, *Vitaceae*
      grape
        brandy
        champagne
        cream of tartar /
        dried "currant"
        raisin
        wine
        wine vinegar
      muscadine
53 Linden Family, *Tiliaceae*
      *basswood (linden)
54 Mallow Family, *Malvaceae*
      *althea root
      cottonseed oil
      *hibiscus (roselle)
      okra
55 Sterculia Family, *Sterculiaceae*
      *chocolate (cacao)
      *cocoa
        cocoa butter
      cola nut
56 Dillenia Family, *Dilleniaceae*
      Chinese gooseberry (kiwi
        berry)
57 Tea Family, *Theaceae*
      *tea
58 Passion Flower Family,
                Passifloraceae
      granadilla (passion fruit)
59 Papaya Family, *Caricaceae*
      papaya
60 Cactus Family, *Cactaceae*
      prickly pear
61 Pomegranate Family, *Puniceae*
      pomegranate
      grenadine
62 Sapucaya Family,
                Lecythidaceae
      Brazil nut
      sapucaya nut (paradise nut)
63 Myrtle Family, *Myrtaceae*
      allspice (*Pimenta*)
      clove
      *eucalyptus
      guava
64 Ginseng Family, *Araliaceae*

      *American ginseng
      *Chinese ginseng
65 Carrot Family,
                Umbelliferae
      angelica
      anise
      caraway
      carrot
        carrot syrup
      celeriac (celery root)
      celery
        *seed & leaf
      chervil
      coriander
      cumin
      dill
        dill seed
      *fennel
        finocchio
          Florence fennel
      *gotu kola
      *lovage
      *parsley
      parsnip
      sweet cicely
66 Heath Family, *Ericaceae*
      *bearberry
      *blueberry
      cranberry
      *huckleberry
67 Sapodilla Family, *Sapotaceae*
      chicle (chewing gum)
68 Ebony Family, *Ebonaceae*
      American persimmon
      kaki (Japanese persimmon)
69 Olive Family, *Oleaceae*
      olive (green or ripe)
        olive oil
70 Morning-Glory Family,
                Convolvulaceae
      sweet potato
71 Borage Family, *Boraginaceae*
      (Herbs)
      borage
      *comfrey (leaf & root)
72 Verbena Family, *Verbenaceae*
      *lemon verbena

73 Mint Family, *Labiatae* (Herbs)
  apple mint
  basil
  bergamot
  *catnip
  *chia seed
  clary
  *dittany
  *horehound
  *hyssop
  lavender
  *lemon balm
  marjoram
  oregano
  *pennyroyal
  *peppermint
  rosemary
  sage
  *spearmint
  summer savory
  thyme
  winter savory
74 Potato Family,
      Solanaceae
  eggplant
  ground cherry
  pepino
    (melon pear)
  pepper (Capsicum)
    bell, sweet
    cayenne
    chili
    paprika
    pimiento
  potato
  tobacco
  tomatillo
  tomato
  tree tomato
75 Pedalium Family,
      Pedaliaceae
  sesame seed
    sesame oil
    tahini
76 Madder Family, *Rubiaceae*
  *coffee
  woodruff

77 Honeysuckle Family,
        Caprifoliaceae
  elderberry
  elderberry flowers
78 Valerian Family, *Valerianaceae*
  corn salad (fetticus)
79 Gourd Family, *Cucurbitaceae*
  chayote
  Chinese preserving melon
  cucumber
  gherkin
  loofah (*Luffa*) (vegetable
    sponge)
  muskmelons
    cantaloupe
    casaba
    crenshaw
    honeydew
    Persian melon
  pumpkin
    pumpkin seed & meal
  squashes
    acorn
    buttercup
    butternut
    Boston marrow
    caserta
    cocozelle
    crookneck & straightneck
    cushaw
    golden nugget
    Hubbard varieties
    pattypan
    turban
    vegetable spaghetti
    zucchini
  watermelon
80 Composite Family, *Compositae*
  *boneset
  *burdock root
  cardoon
  chamomile
  *chicory
  coltsfoot
  costmary
  dandelion
  endive

escarole
globe artichoke
*goldenrod
Jerusalem artichoke
    artichoke flour
lettuce
    celtuce
pyrethrum
romaine
safflower oil
salsify (oyster plant)
santolina (herb)

scolymus (Spanish oyster
    plant)
scorzonera (black salsify)
southernwood
sunflower
    sunflower seed, meal & oil
tansy (herb)
tarragon (herb)
witloof chicory (French
    endive)
wormwood (absinthe)
*yarrow

Animal

81 *Mollusks*
    Gastropods
        abalone
        snail
    Cephalopod
        squid
    Pelecypods
        clam
        cockle
        mussel
        oyster
        scallop
82 *Crustaceans*
    crab
    crayfish
    lobster
    prawn
    shrimp
83 *Fishes (saltwater)*
84 Herring Family
    menhaden
    pilchard (sardine)
    sea herring
85 Anchovy Family
    anchovy
86 Eel Family
    American eel
87 Codfish Family
    cod (scrod)
    cusk
    haddock

    hake
    pollack
88 Sea Catfish Family
    ocean catfish
89 Mullet Family
    mullet
90 Silverside Family
    silverside (whitebait)
91 Sea Bass Family
    grouper
    sea bass
92 Tilefish Family
    tilefish
93 Bluefish Family
    bluefish
94 Jack Family
    amberjack
    pompano
    yellow jack
95 Dolphin Family
    dolphin
96 Croaker Family
    croaker
    drum
    sea trout
    silver perch
    spot
    weakfish (spotted sea trout)
97 Porgy Family
    northern scup (porgy)

116   Diet Planning

CHAPTER 10

Relatively Safe Foods

"GROWN MAN that I was, I stood in the middle of a grocery store and cried like a baby. I was hungry. My billfold was full of money. I was in a grocery store but there was no food I could buy that would not make me ill."

The chemically sensitive man speaking to us, referring to his first experience in a store after his return from the hospital, described one of the most problematical facts of life: There is no guarantee that any food is perfectly safe. Unless you grow your own food, you cannot be sure of its purity. No, we take that back—even your own food can be contaminated by pesticides carried by the wind from neighboring property or by mass spraying from the air.

The roadblocks to finding pure foods are probably the most frustrating aspect of the fight for a return to nontoxic living. When one government agency doesn't hamper us another does with regulations that favor big business. By accident or design? We don't know. You be the judge. Volumes couldn't cover all the stories, so we'll just present one case in point.

You can go into a health food store and buy buffalo meat wrapped in nontoxic butcher paper. That same store cannot carry pork products wrapped in butcher paper. Pork products, the regulations say, must be wrapped in heat-sealed plastic. We wonder if there would be a ban on butcher-paper-wrapped buffalo if the big meat companies began packaging and selling buffalo meat.

Since we can't be sure of "safe" foods, we settle for "relatively safe foods," or, as Dr. Joseph Morgan terms it, "chemically less contaminated." Such foods can be divided into three groups:

Organic. In some states this label is applied to foods grown with only natural fertilizers. Look for labels so marked, stating "no pesticides or preservatives, no hormones injected into the animals, no additives."

Natural. Foods labeled "natural" contain no preservatives or additives, including artificial coloring or artificial flavoring. There are some foods marked "natural" that many sensitive patients can tolerate even though they are not organically grown.

Commercial. There is a limited list of "safe" foods available in commercial markets (see below). But first, here are six food items you should avoid:

Sugar
White flour
White rice
Foods with preservatives (especially BHT and BTA)
Foods with artificial coloring
Foods with artificial flavoring

Many doctors believe that from the evidence they have seen, half of existing health problems would disappear if these six items were avoided. This usually means cooking from scratch, avoiding the great majority of processed foods. (There are some processed foods in health food stores and health food sections of supermarkets that are free from the six items.)

Many local health food stores do not carry a large supply of organically grown fresh produce and meat. However, they usually know local sources. Also, there is a directory of organic food sources listed by state, the *Guide to Organic Food Shopping and Organic Living* (Rodale Press, Emmaus, Pa. 18049). Although the guide is quite reliable, you will have to check each source carefully to be sure of its purity before stocking with a lot of food. Test the food by ordering foods you know you can tolerate. (Many safe foods arrive in unsafe wrappings such as plastic, thus adding contaminants to pure foods. That problem limits the amount of packaged food that can be used by the sensitive person.) *

We have no scientific evidence as proof, but we know that many patients have been able to tolerate meat from the third or fourth generation of animals that have been fed organically and received no hormone injections. You can usually find farmers in your area who practice organic farming.

Another way to get help in obtaining relatively safe foods is through HEAL. As this book goes to press, HEAL is in the process of preparing an outline of procedures for setting up cooperative purchasing for their chapter members. A mini-chapter requires only ten members.

---

* As this goes to press, we are delighted that we have finally communicated our message to one of the leading suppliers—Shiloh Farms of Arkansas. They are in the process of consulting with clinical ecologists to design a series of nontoxic wrappings. They are also preparing a new line of foods that will eventually conform to the rotary diversified diet. We hope that other companies will follow suit.

RELATIVELY SAFE FOODS FROM COMMERCIAL STORES

Avocados, Royal Hawaiian jet-flown pineapple from Hawaii, jicama, macadamia nuts, mandarin oranges from Japan, mangoes, papayas, watercress, frozen Alaskan king crab, frozen South African lobster tails, lamb from New Zealand or Australia, tomato juice bottled in glass.

To help you get started, we're presenting a list of brand names of relatively safe products. You should be aware of the fact that not all these products are organic. However, some of the natural products have been tolerated by patients; test them and see for yourself.

Do Not Accept the Brand Names as Recommendations. Even the most acceptable companies frequently have products that are not safe or that have too many ingredients, representing too many food families.

Erewhon products are tolerated by many people. Their whole-wheat lasagna is made from 100 percent organically grown wheat and is probably safe for anyone who is not wheat-sensitive. Their brown-rice spaghetti is made from organically grown brown rice along with organically grown whole wheat. But someone buying it because of the rice might still be allergic to the wheat. Similarly, Erewhon lists organic spinach powder in some of their pastas. Unless you know the contents of their spinach powder, you can't be sure of the product.

You will find some products marked "unsprayed" as opposed to "organic." For example, one store sold unsprayed peanuts. On checking we found that they rotated crops in the same field, rotating peanuts with cotton. The year that cotton was grown they sprayed, but not when the peanuts were grown the alternating year. It's highly unlikely that the peanuts were uncontaminated.

BRAND NAMES OF RELATIVELY SAFE FOODS

Ahlers
Alta Dena
Arden
Arrowhead Mills

Barbara's Bakery
Biotta
Bonny Tree
Briggs Way
  Salmon

Celestial
  Seasoning
Chico San

Deaf Smith
De Sousa
Dr. Bonner

Elams
El Molino

Erewhon
Escondito

Golden Acres
Good Food
  Brand
Greene Herb
  Gardens herbs
  and spices

Hain's
Hansen
Health Valley
Heinke
Hunza

Jolly Joan

Knudsen

L&A

Mrs. Woods

Natural Nectar
Nordic

Old Colony

Pride of the Farm
Pure and Simple

Red Star

Shiloh Farms

Tree of Life

Walnut Acres

CHAPTER 11

Yeast, Malt, and Molds

EVEN THOUGH you are not allergic to wheat, you may still become ill after eating bread, the culprit very likely being yeast. Some people can drink milkshakes but are allergic to malted milkshakes. Others have no reaction to a meat gravy, but become ill if there are mushrooms (a mold food) in it.

We discuss yeast and molds together because, in a manner of speaking, they are first cousins. Although they are very different in many respects, they are of the same family—the Fungi Family. Therefore, if you are allergic to one, you should be very careful about the foods of the other. Accordingly, when planning your rotary diet, have them both at the same meal—perhaps a yeast food like vinegar and a mold food like cheese or mushrooms.

Dr. Dor W. Brown, Jr., an eye, ear, nose, and throat specialist of Fredericksburg, Texas, conducts a yearly seminar for those in his field who have become convinced, as he is, that they can no longer treat their patients without giving major consideration to foods and inhalants which affect those organs. Since yeast and molds are troublesome for so many people, Dr. Brown prepared a list of foods containing yeast, malt, and mold. With his permission, we have updated his list and tailored it to the needs of this book.

Yeast Additives. The following foods contain yeast as an additive ingredient in preparation (often called leavening or baker's yeast):

Breads: light bread, hamburger buns, hotdog buns, rolls (homemade or canned), crackers, pretzels, canned icebox biscuits.
Pastries: cookies, pies, cakes.
Flour enriched with vitamins from yeast.
Milk fortified with vitamins from yeast.
Meat fried in cracker crumbs or flour.

Pancakes, waffles, muffins, cornbread, and biscuits made with baking powder or soda can be substituted for baker's yeast products. Unbleached 100 percent whole-wheat crackers (matzos) for people who can eat wheat but not yeast are available from Streit's. For distributors in your area write: Aron Streit, Inc.[1]

Yeast-Forming Substances. The following foods contain yeast or yeastlike substances, because of their nature or the nature of their manufacture or preparation (including brewer's and distiller's yeast and malt):

> Vinegars (apple, pear, grape, and distilled), either used as such or in the preparation of catsup, mayonnaise, salad dressings, barbecue sauce, tomato sauce, sauerkraut, horseradish, pickles, olives, mince pie, Gerber's oatmeal, and barley cereal.
>
> Fermented beverages: whiskey, wine, brandy, gin, rum, vodka, beer, root beer.
>
> Fruit juices, either canned or frozen. Only home-squeezed are yeast-free.

Freshly squeezed lemon juice can be used in place of vinegar in mayonnaise.

Yeast Derivatives. The following contain substances that are derived from yeast or yeastlike substances:

> Vitamin B, whether capsule or tablet. Multiple vitamins that contain vitamin B.
>
> Antibiotics; meat from animals that are fed antibiotics.

Malt Products. Cereals, candy, malted milk drinks, and some fermented beverages.

Mold Foods. Mushrooms, truffles, morels.

Mold-Containing Foods. Buttermilk, cheeses of all kinds, including cottage cheese, cream cheese, sour cream, sour-cream butter, condiments, spices, and dried herbs of all kinds (pepper, cinnamon).

Molds (Environmental). (see Chapter 24).

Storage and Handling of Foods

If you are sensitive to mold, do not store fruits and vegetables in your basement regardless of how cold the basement may be. Root vegetables, especially potatoes and carrots, start molding from the time they are taken from the ground. You must be careful to wash root vegetables thoroughly. Better yet, have someone else wash and peel them. The mold-sensitive individual should not eat the peelings of potatoes, carrots, or other root vegetables.

Dr. Marshall Mandell, who has done considerable research on molds, cautions that if you are experiencing fatigue and depression along with a stuffy nose, runny eyes, asthma, and mental confusion, it would be wise to be checked for mold sensitivity.

Warning: Antibiotics derived from mold should be approached with caution.[2] If an individual gets more of an antibiotic than he can tolerate, it could result in damage to the eighth cranial nerve, which has to do with hearing and balance. This raises an interesting question: If people can react severely to the occasional use of an antibiotic because they are allergic to mold, how much damage is resulting from their daily or frequent consumption of mold foods such as cheese?

PART III
CREATIVE COOKING

CHAPTER 12

Introduction to Creative Cooking

D R. LAWRENCE DICKEY, a firm advocate of the rotary diversified diet believes that whenever a patient has improved for a couple of years and then had a reversal in the state of his health, the major cause was almost certain to be the failure to remain on this diet.[1]

One food at a time is the healthiest approach for the acutely food sensitive person. This section on creative cooking is prepared for those who wish to deviate a little by eating a greater variety of foods but still wish to use the rotation system. It is also prepared with prevention in mind. For those of you who have no known allergies or food addictions but wish to prevent them, this section will be helpful in planning interesting meals that will follow a rotation diet.

Once the rotary diet has been stabilized, you can begin to experiment. You can introduce multiple-food meals and you can plan for variety, nutrition, and taste. Although it is advised that rotation be continued, some people choose to break the rotation habit during holiday or vacation periods and do so without ill effects; others prefer to adhere strictly to the method of eating which returned them to a functioning state of health.

Rotating Multiple Food Meals

For those who continue to rotate foods in their diet, the concept, with a few exceptions, remains the same. The main difference is the management of multiple-food meals. As they are introduced, you should try to use foods of the same family at the same meal: a stew using celery, carrots, and/or parsley; a sauce using green peppers and tomatoes; a pie using cherries and almonds. If they are not eaten at the same meal, the foods in the same family should be separated by four days.

Herbs and Oils. It is important to rotate herbs and oils. If almonds are used as a pie crust, almond oil should also be used; corn oil should be used for a meal in which corn is eaten; soy or peanut oil for the meal using legumes (peanuts, soybeans, peas).

Balancing the Diet. The first thing to be considered is animal protein.

The ideal plan would include use of mammals, fish, fowl, amphibians, and crustaceans, a large enough variety to eat animal proteins once or twice a day. If this is not possible, a good substitute is vegetable protein (nuts, seeds).

The second consideration is fruits and vegetables. If possible, each day's menu should include fruit, a green vegetable, and a yellow vegetable. On a day in which grains and starches cannot be used, choose a vegetable high in carbohydrates such as potatoes or sweet potatoes.*

Avoiding Sugar

Ideally, it is best to avoid all sweeteners, including honey and syrup. We have included recipes using honey and syrup only because they are less harmful than sugar and some people may prefer to diminish their sweet intake gradually. We recommend that each time you use one of these recipes you decrease the quantity of the sweetener. After six or eight months without sweets your bad habit will be broken. You will find you will prefer the natural flavor, and you no longer need to risk the harmful effects of sugars. A word of caution—you cannot break the habit of adding sweeteners if you continue using them even in small amounts. Eventually you must abstain totally.

* For food value tables see Catherine Elwood's *Feel Like a Million*, pages 328–344.[2]
The professional is referred to the publication by the Department of Agriculture.[3]

CHAPTER 13

Cooking Hints

AIRING FOODS. According to Dr. Kailin, foods wrapped in plastic are penetrated by the molecules of the plastic. If you have to tear the plastic to open the package, you know that it has been heat sealed, and there is no way of clearing that food of the molecules.

If the top has been secured by the use of a wire twist, you can open the package without breaking the seal. It is then probable that most of the plastic residue can be aired from the food in a matter of three or four days. Dr. Kailin has suggested that the airing time for food stored in plastic can be cut from three days to one or two, by putting the food in a covered glass jar containing a charcoal filter.

If the food is a wet solid, put it in an open glass jar and place this in a larger jar which contains charcoal. Cover the larger jar.

Banana Storage. Since it is difficult to get ungassed bananas (gassing is used to ripen bananas artifically), when they are available buy them in large quantities and store in the home, using as they ripen. Freeze the excess before it spoils to keep on hand for banana cakes, banana shakes, or banana sundaes.

Chopping Boards. Wooden chopping boards and tables are not recommended because it is impossible to insure against the formation of bacteria. In addition, invisible food particles would interfere with rotating foods. Use Corningware chopping boards.

Cleaning Foods. When washing large quantities of fruits, vegetables, meat, or fish, conserve spring water by using a large roasting pan to hold the water.

Combining Foods. When cooking in quantity, use only one food at a time. Combine foods only when they are defrosted and ready to eat. You may need to change rotation or may become allergic to a food once considered safe.

Cooktop Range. There have been good reports on the Corningware Cooktop range. There is no odor and it is very clean. Many feel this stove top is an improvement over regular electric stoves, which give off fumes at high temperatures from formaldehyde coating on the surface underneath the burners, creosote-coated wires, and fiberglass insulation.

Fish. Whenever you buy fish from *any* source, check the packing box, which must be labeled if antibiotics have been used.

Freezing Fruits. It is more wholesome and more pleasurable to eat fruits when they are fresh. However, with the increasing cost of fruits and specifically, organic fruits, it is wise to buy them in quantity at the height of their season and freeze them. Canning is not recommended unless there is a shortage of freezing space, because the heating process destroys so much of the nutrient value of the food.

It is necessary to acquire a taste for certain defrosted, frozen fruits, for example, bananas. Many people have told us that they enjoy them when still partially frozen. Frozen fruit, when placed in a blender and mixed with a juice, makes a delicious fruit shake.

Wash and freeze whole: apples, apricots, blueberries, cherries, grapes, peaches, pears, persimmons, plums. (If apples, peaches, or pears have been cut first, dip in brine solution made with sea salt and well water to prevent discoloring.)

Peel and remove seeds or core: pineapple, melons (cantaloupe, Crenshaw, honeydew, muskmelon, and watermelon). Divide oranges into sections.

Gamey Taste. To remove gamey taste from wild game or the fowl taste and odor from fowl, use kosher salt (a coarse sea salt available at Jewish delicatessens or in some large food markets). After soaking meat for thirty minutes in spring water, place the meat on a steel or chrome rack over the sink and cover each piece liberally with the salt. Let stand for one hour; rinse with spring water. Cook as desired.

Gravy. It is desirable to use gravy for the added flavor it gives to meats and/or vegetables and because the meat extracts contain creatine, an energy-important molecule. When making gravy, if it dries brown and adheres to the sides and bottom of the pan, add a little water to the pan and with a spoon gently scrape it off until the water turns a golden brown. Too much water makes the gravy tasteless. If the gravy congeals in the pan, add a little water, heat gently, and pour into a jar. When cool, the fat on top can easily be removed if desired.

Herb Salts. To make herb salts (celery salt, onion salt) blend a given volume of preblended dried herbs with an equal volume of sea salt. (Blending of herbs changes the volume.)

Herbs. To dry herbs, tie in loose bunches and hang in a shady, well-ventilated room until dry. An alternative method is to put herbs in a very slow oven, not over 130° F. Parsley takes two hours, other herbs around one hour. Crush dried herbs to powder with rolling pin. Pack in airtight containers and label. Dry seeds by spreading evenly on thin cloth rack. Dry in sun, turning daily.

Low Temperature Cooking. Some patients have been experimenting with low-temperature cooking as suggested by Adele Davis, because many chemically sensitive persons react when fats are subjected to high temperatures. The fats split into glycerol and the glycerol into toxic Acrolein. (Dr. Alsop Corwin reports that the browned surface of seared meats and caramelized sugar, as on glazed ham, contain substances which are carcinogenic.[1] He favors cooking food slowly so as not to produce browning or charring.)

Hot Drink. Combine ¾ cup boiling water with ¼ cup tolerated juice.

Iron. Cast-iron frying pans can be used to add iron to the diet.

Lemon. When using half a lemon remember the blossom end (the furthest part from the stem) is the sweetest part of the fruit.

Marinating. Lemon juice can be substituted for vinegar for marinating meats or fish, in mayonnaise, and in oil salad dressing.

Method. Cover pots to keep air away from food while cooking. Do not beat air into foods.

Motors. To avoid problems with ozone given off by the electric motors of cooking implements (blenders, mixers, food processors) try to have plenty of fresh air in the cooking area. Make frequent trips away from the area where appliances are being used. When possible, use these appliances on a patio or terrace.

Oil. Use pure oils, not blends. Use a pure safflower oil or a pure sesame oil or a pure almond oil. It is also advisable that you use cold, unpressed oils. One or two tablespoons of such a pure oil poured over chopped, raw vegetables with a little salt makes a very interesting salad. If you are using sesame seed oil on a salad, add sesame seeds; if you are using sunflower seed oil, add sunflower seeds to enhance the taste and nutritional value. If you are steaming a vegetable, when it is ready to serve pour a little bit of the oil over it to improve the flavor.

Oven. Those sensitive to metals should try doing all oven cooking in a stove kept in the basement to reduce the period of exposure to the heated metal. Top of stove units cause allergic problems when set on higher temperatures. Try using a Corningware electric skillet.

Parsley. To store fresh parsley, place in a jar with stems immersed in one or two inches of water. Leaves should not touch the water. Parsley will stay fresh for days in a capped jar in the refrigerator.

Paper Towels. Don't use paper towels to dry food; they are made of bleached, treated wood pulp. Use cotton toweling instead.

Raw Cashew Nuts. When roasted, cashews may produce no reaction, but raw they contain a shell oil similar to the oleoresin that produces the rash from poison plants. So if you are allergic to poison ivy, poison oak, or poison sumac, the chances are you are allergic to raw cashews and should not eat them without being tested by a doctor for a reaction.

Salt. We recommend only sea salt. One of the purest products available is DeSousa solar evaporated salt, a rock salt which requires the use of only half as much as other salt. For salt grinder, see Walnut Acres catalog.

School Lunches. Prepare standard hot meal in Dine-out cartons (see below), freeze them. Remove and have your child take to school for warming up in the oven at lunchtime. One mother sends a one-week supply on Monday to be kept in the school freezer. Permission must be granted by school authorities.

Sesame Seeds. Sesame seeds are one of the few vegetable proteins that contain methianine, the amino acid that is missing from grains and legumes. Therefore, such things as beans cooked with sesame seeds form a complete protein.

Shrimp. To cook, use a stainless steel steamer inside a stainless steel pot with a tight-fitting cover. (This cuts down tremendously on the unpleasant cooking smell.) The shrimp should be laid on the steamer over ½" of spring water, and cooked in a single layer. It takes only a few minutes of steaming to cook them through; you need comparatively little water.

Soda. Try to limit the use of soda in cooking and baking; it destroys valuable food properties.

Soup. Save cooking water which is rich in nutrients for use in soups and gravies.

Storage. One-gallon glass jars with wide mouths make wonderful storage for fresh fruits and vegetables in the refrigerator. Totally airtight, well-washed produce keeps for weeks without spoilage.

Stove Hood. Use especially when preparing food to which anyone in the house is allergic. Get the kind which is vented to the outside, not just the charcoal trap kind.

Sweeten-to-Taste. When this phrase appears in a recipe, avoid sugars and liquid sweeteners. Instead, blend in fresh or dried fruit of your choice. We have had good results with bananas, coconut, dates, figs, or raisins.

Vinegar. Use a vinegar made from a tolerated food (grapes, apples). Do not rotate vinegars. No matter what food it is derived from, it is a yeast and must be treated as such. For those sensitive to apples and wheat, use an inexpensive Spanish white wine vinegar. Remove the cork and put it back on lightly; let stand a few months. When the vinegar is ready, add 2 tablespoons to a new bottle of wine to make vinegar in a two-week period.

Walnut Acres. Mail order house supplier of foods.[2] Write for their catalog; read it carefully. Only some of their products meet our standards. We object to their use of plastic wrappings and plasticized metal cans and their multiple-ingredient products. Only some of their foods are organic. However, they usually label their foods carefully. If you have any questions, they are cooperative, and trustworthy.

Water. Water can become moldy. To reuse the same bottles for well or spring water, it is wise to sterilize the bottles and the caps from time to time. Place gallon-size bottles, uncapped, in the oven at 250° F. for 1½ hours. Boil the caps for twenty minutes. (The top shelf of the oven can be used simultaneously for low-heat cooking.)

Wrapping. Pure cellophane rolls may be obtained from paper distributors such as Zellerback Paper Co. or Blake, Moffitt, and Towne. For cellophane bags write Nuvita Food Company.[3] Available in one-half, one, two, three, four, five and ten-pound sizes.

Snack-size Dine-out cartons, #906, with inside aluminum coating, may be obtained from American Can Company.[4] The two-pound cellophane bag fits into this snugly. (The aluminum is not recommended for direct contact with food because most aluminum is contaminated either from the oil of the rollers used to make it or because the aluminum has been plasticized). The cartons stack neatly in the freezer and can be used over and over again. For storing larger quantities of food, use the E-Z foil freezer containers (available in supermarkets). The four- or five-pound size cellophane bag fits into these boxes. They also stack easily in the freezer.

For Mason jars that now use plastic lids, cut a circle of cellophane the size of the lid and place between lid and top of jar.

Wrapping Food. Do not store food in plastic. Also avoid aluminum foil if possible. Under no circumstances should heated food be wrapped in plastic or aluminum. An even more dangerous practice is cooking food or heating food in aluminum or plastic, for example, disposable, soft plastic liners for infants' nursing bottles.

To avoid freezer burn when freezing, store chickens and large cuts of meat in cellophane bags. After sealing them with a twist, double-wrap in butcher paper or aluminum foil (as long as the foil does not touch the food). For turkeys and roasts too big for the bag, wrap first in cellophane roll paper and then rewrap in butcher paper. If you are wrapping more than one piece of meat, place a piece of cellophane paper between the pieces.

CHAPTER 14

Substitutions

THIS CHAPTER deals with two kinds of substitutions: Those for persons with multiple allergies who find it virtually impossible to use recipes without some substitutions, and those that can be eaten for starch content when grains and potatoes must be avoided.

WARNING: SUGAR SUBSTITUTIONS

So much has been discovered about the danger of sugar that we have omitted all recipes containing it. Although most doctors involved with nutrition recommend that honey be avoided as well, for those who must use a sweetener, tupelo or sage honey is suggested.

The following guideline will also be given at the beginning of the *Cookbook for the Allergic Person* but it bears repeating:

Sugar Substitute

1. One-half cup of honey equals 1 cup sugar.
2. Deduct ¼ cup liquid from recipe when using honey in place of sugar.

STARCH SUBSTITUTIONS FOR GRAIN-FREE, WHITE POTATO-FREE DIETS

Arrowroot Flour (Starch). Use for cookies, to thicken fruit juice to pudding consistency, to thicken meat sauce or gravy.

Artichoke. Available as a flour.

Avocado. High in calories.

Banana. Slice into citrus or pineapple juice. Make cereal with banana flakes (baby counter in the supermarket). Baked in oven, it is good with chicken. Buy green plantain (Puerto Rico grows it) and broil thin slices brushed with oil, mash when soft, and broil again to make a "banana chip."

Buckwheat. Buckwheat flour may be used in pancakes, groats as hot cereal. If you are allergic to wheat, do not use buckwheat more than once every two weeks as an allergy to it develops easily.

134

Ground Nuts and Seeds. Use to make fruit cake. Pumpkin or sunflower seeds make good snacks.

Lima or Navy Beans, Green Peas. Use for lentil soup, pork and beans, split pea soup. Lima bean flour is available and can be used to make bread.

Ñame, Malanga, Yuca. These are starchy tubers which can be cooked and eaten like white potato. Tropical potato is another root prepared the same way.

Pancakes. See recipes.

Snack Foods. Nuts, dates, figs, raisins, dried fruits such as apple, peach, apricot. (Tend to produce intestinal gas—go easy.)

Soy Bean. Flour is used in pancakes, muffins, cookies, waffles. Note: Processed soy flour contains wheat.

Sweet Potato. Use boiled, mashed, baked, steamed, or candied.

Tapioca. Use tapioca starch to thicken fruit juices. Soak pearl tapioca overnight, then cook it with fruit juice. Use tapioca starch for puddings, cookies, cake.

Winter Squash. Hubbard, butternut, acorn squash are good examples. Pumpkin is similar in its uses.

SUBSTITUTE FOODS FOR THE GRAIN-SENSITIVE PERSON

The grain-sensitive patient who is also unable to use white potato can obtain substitute foods at Spanish or Puerto Rican food markets.

Yuca. Properly called cassava, yuca is a fleshy protuberance on the roots of a small tree, from which tapioca is made. Peel off the coarse, stringy bark with a table knife so that you get into the yellow layer between the bark and the white flesh of the tuber. The tuber may then be quartered and boiled like a potato. The raw tuber may be made into a biscuit-like bread substitute called "bammy." To make bammy: Grate the peeled raw yuca on the finest cheese grater obtainable. Squeeze the wet gratings through a clean towel to remove excess moisture. Toss the moist meal through a colander to fluff it up. Salt if desired. Place in a heavy frying pan without added fat or oil. The rims used to hold Mason jar lids in place are convenient forms for small bammy cakes. Fill about ½" deep, or make a large single pancake. Cook at medium high heat about four minutes. The vegetable gum melts, turns a little gray and holds the particles of meal together. At this point flip the cake over and brown the other side. Eat like toast or use as a pancake. Can be stored for several days.

Ñame. A large smooth-barked tuber which can be peeled, cut in pieces, and cooked like white potato. For those sensitive to tapioca, the following bammy can be made with ñame:

Peel. Grate finely. Add salt to taste (do not squeeze in towel). Place in oiled cake pan in oven, filling about ½″ to ¾″ deep. Bake at 350° F. about thirty minutes, turning once ten minutes before finishing. Use as a pancake. Clove, nutmeg, grated orange peel, or cinnamon can be added for variety.

Food to Be Replaced	Measure	Substitution	Directions and Comments
Baking Powder	1 teaspoon	½ teaspoon cream of tartar	Notice that there are three formulas stated here. In
	1 teaspoon	¼ teaspoon baking soda	each case there is a single-action baking powder which begins to rise the
	1 teaspoon	1 teaspoon cream of tartar ½ teaspoon baking soda	moment it contacts liquid (acid). A double-action powder also rises and then has a second rise caused
		1¾ teaspoons cream of tartar ½ teaspoon baking soda	by oven heat. Since single action does not have a second rise, to have maximum rise, add to liquid ingredients as late as possible, and work quickly. Of the three formulae, the larger the amount of baking soda, the greater the loss of nutrients but the greater the rise.
Bread Crumbs for meat loaf and patties		Cooked oatmeal Grated nuts Grated potato or other starchy vegetable Grated cauliflower for dieters	
Butter	1 cup	1 cup milk ¾ cup water ¼ cup oil, egg, or gelatin	The egg replaces protein.
	1 cup	⅞ cup oil ½ teaspoon salt	Oil pie crust is easier to press into pan with finger or spoon rather than roll it.

Food to Be Replaced	Measure	Substitution	Directions and Comments
	1 cup	1 cup animal fat	Pork fat is soft, easy to handle. Lard makes finest of all pastry crust. Beef fat tends to be stiff. Lamb fat is quite stiff—good in candy and cakes that tend to be heavy.
	1 cup	1 cup poultry fat	Chicken fat is fine. Goose and duck are softer. See "Cooking Hints," Chapter 13 (rendering fat).
Chocolate or Cocoa	1 tablespoon	1 tablespoon carob flour	
Chocolate, melted	1 ounce	3 tablespoons carob 1½ tablespoons oil	Heat until melted.
Coffee or Tea	1 cup	Herb tea	
Coffee Cream	1 cup	⅛ cup milk 3 tablespoons creamery butter	Use blender.
Corn Meal		Millet Potato meal Soy flour	
Cream, heavy	1 cup	¾ cup milk ⅓ cup butter	Use blender.
Eggs	1 egg	½ teaspoon baking powder 2 tablespoons flour ½ tablespoon fat	Eggs are used in cooking for purposes other than nutrition. The yolks add flavor and oil (richness). They hold a cooked product together. They can be beaten to hold air bubbles and so add lightness to cakes, cookies, and puddings. Choose a substitute with these functions in mind.
	1 egg	2 tablespoons water 1 tablespoon oil 2 tablespoons baking powder	
	1 egg	2 tablespoons water 2 teaspoons baking powder	

Food to Be Replaced	Measure	Substitution	Directions and Comments
Eggs (cont.)	1 egg yolk	½ teaspoon baking powder 2 tablespoons flour	One formula calls for 2 teaspoons baking powder for the first egg in a cake recipe and 1 teaspoon baking powder for each additional egg.
	1 egg white	½ tablespoon fat 1 tablespoon baking powder 4 tablespoons flour	
		Apple or other fruit sauce. Cooked starchy vegetable puree. Flaxseed-water mixture. Cottage cheese Sour milk Nut butter	For body and stickiness.
	1 egg	1 teaspoon baking powder Grated yuca	Gives rising power but won't hold (lacks body and stickiness).
	1 egg in cookies	3 tablespoons pureed fruit	Using thick pureed fruit helps hold and adds good flavor—gives a chewy cookie.
	1 egg in puddings	Gelatin— 1 tablespoon to 2 cups milk or less	Soak gelatin in ¼ cup liquid (cold) and stir into hot liquid until dissolved. Allow to cool and thicken (not solidify—warm up if it does set) and then beat (rotary beater) until light and bubbly.
Flour, White		Whole wheat	In pie crust (oil type) the whole-wheat product will not roll well. Put the ball of dough into the pie pan and press it into place using your fingers. Whole-wheat flour in cookies and

Food to be replaced	Measure	Substitution	Directions and Comments
			baking powder biscuits will give a smaller, dark-colored product with good flavor. The biscuits will be heavier.
Flour, Wheat		Rye, Other flours	Rye makes a stiff, sticky dough, slow to rise. Only wheat and rye have enough gluten to hold a rise; other flours are likely to make a heavy, moist product. When using them, do not open oven door (makes draft), do not jar the oven. Allow to cool gradually before handling.
	1 cup flour	1 cup nuts, ground	For pie crust, add a little salt. For easy handling add 1 tablespoon or more of oil and use fingers or spoon to press into pan. May be used as a flour substitute in meat loaf. For cookies, add salt and enough thick fruit puree or sauce to hold cookies together. Whole nutmeats, when grated, are dry; when ground, oily; when blended, floury.
Flour, Whole Wheat	1 cup	¾ cup corn meal	
	1 cup	½ cup oatmeal finely ground	
Flours for thickener		Arrowroot starch Artichoke flour Barley flour Buckwheat flakes, Buckwheat Poi Potato flour	

Food to Be Replaced	Measure	Substitution	Directions and Comments
Flours for thickener (cont.)		Potato starch Rice flour Tapioca flour or starch	
		Cooked puree of starchy vegetable Shredded raw starchy vegetable	Suggested are carrots, potatoes, parsnips, young turnips, artichokes, squash, kohlrabi, sweet potatoes.
Grain	1 tablespoon wheat flour	½ tablespoon other starch	Other starch can be cornstarch, arrowroot, tapioca, rice, rye, oat, or potato.
	1 cup wheat	4–5 cups bean flour	To obtain bean flour, run dried beans (any kind allowed), a handful at a time, through a blender. Product will be heavier, more moist, and there will be a flavor change. May have to decrease liquid, so be careful in adding.
Milk		Soy bean flour	Mix 1 quart (4 cups) soy bean flour with 1 quart water, gradually to avoid lumping. Strain in cloth bag. Heat drippings in double boiler, stirring often. Refrigerate.
		Spring water Vegetable water Fruit juice	Potato water does not mix well with flour in a sauce or gravy. Use other vegetable water or plain water. Add a little salt and maybe some oil or fat for flavor. Baked goods will be less high, less rich. If using baking powder, do not neutralize the baking powder, thereby reducing rise. Work fast.

Food to Be Replaced	Measure	Substitution	Directions and Comments
Milk (cont.)		Fruit juice	In working with yeast the juice may slow down yeast activity.
		Fruit puree	Especially good in cookies.
		Goat's milk Nut or seed milk	Overnight, soak ½ cup of nuts or seeds in 1 cup liquid (water or juice). Blend to paste. Mix paste with enough liquid for required consistency. Use blender.
	1 cup	⅓ cup dry milk plus water to make 1 cup	
		soy beans	Soak 1½ pounds dried soy beans in spring water for 12 hours. Drain. While grinding in a grinder, pour a slow steady stream of water, making a volume of 1 gallon (4 quarts). Heat to 131° F. Put into clean cloth bag and allow to drip. Heat drippings in double boiler for 45 minutes, stirring often. Sweeten to taste. Add enough water to make 5 quarts. Refrigerate.
		Artichoke Milk: Artichoke flour ½ cup 2 cups water	Mix with electric beater, bring to a boil and simmer for 20 minutes. Drink plain or sweeten to taste.
		Coconut Milk: 1 cup fresh coconut chunks plus its own milk or 1 cup coconut meal 2 cups water	Whip in blender until pulp is fine (or meal is dissolved). Store in a covered jar in the refrigerator.

Food to Be Replaced	Measure	Substitution	Directions and Comments
Milk (cont.)		Nut Milk: ½ cup nuts 1¼ cups cold water	In blender.
		Soy Milk: 1 cup soy flour 4 cups water	Blend ingredients in top of a double boiler. Let stand 2 hours. Place over hot water and bring to a boil (the milk). Cook 20 minutes. Cool and strain. (Leftover flour residue may be added to batters.) Sweeten to taste.
		Sunflower Seed Milk: 1 cup shelled sunflower seeds 3½ cups water	Soak overnight. In blender, blend until you have a white milk and seeds are reduced to pulp. Pour into a fine wire strainer or strain through a thin cloth.
Salad Dressing		Sea salt Oil Lemon juice or vinegar	Use singly or combined as in a French dressing (¼ cup lemon juice or vinegar, ¾ cup oil, ½ teaspoon salt, pinch of herbs, blend.)
		Eggless mayonnaise	See recipes, Part VI.
Vanilla Extract		Vanilla beans	Substitute ¼ teaspoon dried ground vanilla bean for teaspoon vanilla extract. Or place a vanilla bean in a quart jar filled with flour. Leave it for at least a week—the longer the better. Use in place of separate vanilla and flour.
Vinegar		1. Lemon Juice	
		2. Homemade vinegar	See "Cooking Hints," Chapter 13.

CHAPTER 15

Cooking in Large Quantities

PERSONS WITH the chemical susceptibility syndrome report that what they miss most is the convenience of commercially packaged foods. Without these foods how can a patient throw together a fast meal? Nevertheless, you don't have to be a slave to the kitchen because of food allergies. It may not be so easy as going to the market for frozen and canned foods, but it can be done by cooking in large quantities and freezing in meal-size packages.

Reasons. Convenience—fast meals after a hard day's work or when the patient is busy or tired or too ill to cook; money saving—buying in quantities in height of season when cheapest; availability—cooking and storing seasonal foods when they can be purchased; time saving —it takes only twice as long to prepare food for twelve as it does food for one. Freeze eleven extra portions and merely heat when ready to eat.

Since the chemically sensitive individual should not use plastic-coated or aluminum pots, he may have to start from scratch. Where expense is not a consideration, the most desirable pots are cast iron covered with baked enamel; the next preference is Corningware or Pyrex. For the least expensive collection, the following is suggested:

Freezer and Utensils

Here is a beginner's list of things you will need to shop for, if you don't have them already. At first glance the items on this list might appear essential only for the extremely sensitive individual. However, the following case will dispel that notion. A woman, otherwise healthy, discovered that she often began to cough after eating, but could never pinpoint the cause. She felt that foods were not the problem because she could tolerate raw carrots, for example, but was distressed when they were cooked. She was right—it was not the carrots, but rather the aluminum saucepan in which she cooked them. A Christmas gift of Corningware pans led to the discovery that carrots cooked in the new pans did not cause any difficulty.

143

Freezer, the bigger the better. A 6.5-cubic foot costs about as much as a 12-cubic foot. A 15-cubic-foot chest model is just a little more than a 12-cubic-foot upright. A chest type holds much more because shelves on the upright restrict loading; however we prefer the convenience of the upright.

Enamel roasting pan, the biggest that will fit into your oven.

Enamel canner for cooking large cuts, such as a fresh ham.

Twelve-quart enamel pot for steaming vegetables with Marvel steamer.

Two five-quart Dutch ovens, enamel-coated cast iron or Corningware.

Marvel or similar stainless steel steamer.

One or two Corningware chopping boards, 16" × 20".

Large chopping knives, stainless steel with wooden handles.

Four Pyrex cake dishes, recommended size, 13½" × 8¾" × 1¾".

Vegetable brush, natural bristle, wooden handle.

Labels. Use plain freezer tape or self-adhesive labels. Larger labels needed for multiple foods.

Poultry scissors.

Meat thermometer.

Nut cracker.

Parchment paper or cellophane rolls, cellophane bags. For source see *Wrapping* in Chapter 13, p. 133.

Dine-out cartons. For source see *Wrapping* in Chapter 13, p. 133.

Blender. Osterizer has the least amount of plastic and is easiest to clean. The eight- or ten-speed models are unnecessary; a three-speed model is satisfactory.

Mason freezing jars. Wide mouth.

Four Pyrex pie dishes and Pyrex custard dishes for heating frozen foods.

Methods

1. Fast chopping. Use long-handled, long-bladed, very sharp knife with a blade wider than the handle. Thus, when the cutting edge meets the board, there is room for fingers. Example: Place three very thin or two medium carrots side by side. With very firm strokes cut three slices at a time, or with one carrot use fast chopping stroke. At first the slices may be uneven but with a little practice you can chop a pound in the time it takes to slice three carrots with a paring knife—and no more blisters, no more sliver cuts.

2. Fast packaging. Measure cellophane for size. Clear large table space. Place six to nine pieces on table. Ladle out portion desired. Fold, seal and label.

3. Fast folding. Fold paper in half. On three open sides make two folds ½" thick to make a bag. Place the food about 2" from the top of the fold. Bring up bottom edge to meet top edge and fold, crease twice in ½" folds, and seal with Scotch tape or freezer tape.

Turn the paper so that one of the open ends faces you. Fold twice and crease in ½" folds. Then hold the package with the remaining open end in your hand. Gently shake food to the bottom. Fold over as many times as needed to drive out the air and have a solid package. Seal. Box in Dine-out carton and label.

4. You may find it even faster to use two-pound cellophane bags. Leaving enough space for a twist fastener, these fit snugly into a Dine-out carton.

EXAMPLES OF QUANTITY COOKING

Vegetables. Set up an assembly line with one area each for six steps: (1) washing, (2) peeling (when necessary), (3) slicing, (4) steaming, (5) rapid cooling, (6) packaging. Work with one pound at a time. While the first pound is steaming, wash, peel, and slice second pound. Remove first pound from steam, dip into iced, pure drinking water and place in bowl to drain. Steam second pound. Wash, peel, and slice third pound. Package first pound. Remove second pound from steam and start over again.

Preparing ten pounds or more at a time is the greatest time saver. Many extra pounds can be prepared, using the same water and utensils. Quantity preparation gives one a sense of accomplishment and there are supplies ahead for many meals to come.

Meat. Buy a whole fresh ham or equally large piece of meat with bone, have it cut into two pieces. If you're uncertain of the source of the meat remove as much fat as possible. Place in canner, covering meat completely with spring water, about two gallons. Cover the canner.

Place your pot with meat and water on a medium-size burner. Before it reaches the boiling stage, reduce heat to low for one hour so the meat will not toughen. Let the meat simmer until it is fork tender. Remove the meat. Remove the cover from the canner and allow the soup with the bone still in it to simmer down to ⅔ or even ½ the original amount, depending upon the strength of the stock desired. If the meat is not pure organic meat, it is not safe to eat the fat. While the meat is still hot, remove the remaining fat. Package in meal-size portions in cellophane, box in Dine-out cartons, cool in refrigerator and then freeze.

Remove bones from soup, strain, transferring soup to twelve-quart pot for easier refrigeration. Cool overnight in refrigerator or until fat film forms on top. Remove the fat film and discard if the meat was not organic. With organic meat, the fat film can be packaged individually, frozen, and used for seasoning whenever you are cooking with that kind of meat. Fill freezer jars. Label and freeze.

When ready to use, combine meat, soup, and vegetables for meal ready in ten minutes, once soup is defrosted enough to remove from jar. Liquid (frozen in glass) takes longer to defrost than frozen meat. Remember to remove your jar of frozen soup the night before and place in refrigerator. Frozen meat or vegetables can be removed from their package in the frozen state and placed in the saucepan with the defrosted soup.

Note: Do not salt meats until heated and ready to eat. Cooking with salt removes valuable nutrients from food.

Baking Fish. Wash fish thoroughly. Use the top of a roasting pan to rinse the fish with spring water. Two Pyrex cake dishes (13½" × 8¾" × 1¾") will fit on one oven shelf, so the average oven with two shelves accommodates four dishes at a time. Each dish holds about two three-pound fish. Cut fish into serving portions and wrap. Freeze. When ready to eat, remove from the package, place in a Pyrex dish or a Corningware saucepan, and heat in the oven. Or, when going out, remove from the freezer and place in the refrigerator. The fish will be defrosted by the time you return and are ready to eat. It can be eaten unheated. (Many people prefer fish hot from the oven. Fine—if there is time. If the patient must go to work, or if he is not up to cooking, it is good to have a supply of cold fish ready.)

Sweet Potatoes. Wash and cut tops from enough sweet potatoes to fill two cookie sheets. Place in oven preheated to 450°. Remove from oven ten minutes before potatoes are done (thirty-five to fifty minutes, depending on size.) While still very warm, remove skins, slice, wrap, label. If the potatoes are not too large they can be frozen in their skins.

When reheating remember the extra ten minutes needed for thorough baking. Although it takes longer and uses more equipment, the preferred way of cooking sweet potatoes, or any vegetable for that matter, is by steaming.

Lemons. Since organic lemons are not always available, buy them by the dozen when they are plentiful and most reasonable. Squeeze enough to fill one or two ice cube trays. After freezing forty-eight hours, remove from tray and place in glass freezer jar. During scarce season (or when in a hurry) remove one cube and return the rest to freezer. Some vitamin C is lost, but the taste is good.

Nuts. Freeze in shell or remove shell first. Shelling saves space in freezer. Frozen nuts can last two years. Freeze the nuts in Dine-out cartons or glass jars. For those who are lucky enough to be able to use them, nuts are an excellent source of protein, calcium, and energy.

When grinding nuts, seeds, or coconuts for pies, grind a couple of quarts at a time to avoid using the blender every time a pie is made. Keep the ground nuts in the freezer.

Flours and Starch. Do not be afraid to buy these in large quantities. Freeze for forty-eight hours and defrost. They will then keep for months in a tightly capped glass container.

Bananas. Buy green bananas by the dozen when available. Eat them as they ripen but when they will no longer keep, peel, slice and place in blender, first at low, then at high speed. Freeze in pint jars. When leaving the house, remove from freezer and take to work. When ready to eat, combine with chopped nuts. Bananas taste best when defrosted just enough to be edible.

Freeze peeled, very ripe, whole bananas. When ready to eat, defrost only enough to slice. Nuts on cold bananas make a wonderful substitute for an ice cream sundae.

Green bananas may be steamed and served like boiled potatoes. They are starchy rather than sweet.

CHAPTER 16

Basic Methods

MEAT

Use organically grown meats as your first choice. If you can't afford them and must compromise, buy your meats at your regular market but be selective, getting lean meat or meat from grass-fed animals in order to reduce the intake of additives. Avoid pre-packaged meat.

Whenever possible, avoid meats that come from animals that have been injected with hormones and antibiotics. Remove as much fat as possible before cooking, so that it does not melt and become absorbed by the meat. Most of the pesticides are in the fatty part of the meat, including the marbling between meat fibers. Antibiotics are more generally distributed and can't be avoided.

The cooking method selected depends upon three considerations:

Tenderness of Meat. Muscles used often are less tender, have little fat, and have more connective tissue. They increase in flavor with the age of the animal. Muscles that are least exercised are tenderer, more delicate in flavor, juicier, and are fatter in the older animal and leaner in the younger.

Size of Piece. Is it a large chunk? Or is it in small pieces or slices?

How Well Done Should It Be? Beef or lamb are often served rare or medium rare; this is safe only if the meat has been frozen solidly. Pork, veal, and poultry should be well done.

Tender meats are best cooked by dry heat: oven-roasting, oven-broiling, and pan-broiling. Less tender meats are best cooked by moist heat: liquid cooking. In any case, meat cooked at a low temperature will be tenderer, have less shrinkage, be more flavorful (and nourishing), and there will be no burned pan drippings.

Boiling. "Boiled" meat is "simmered" meat; the temperature of the liquid should never go above 185° F. A higher temperature makes the meat stringy, dry, and tough. Do not salt meat until ready to serve.

Roasting. Defrost meat in the refrigerator for at least twenty-four

148

hours before placing it in a preheated oven at 325° F. Place meat, fat side up (that is, formerly fat), uncovered, on a rack in an open, low-sided pan. Do not sear or add water. Insert a meat thermometer in thickest part of meat, being careful not to touch a bone, until it reaches the temperature for the desired degree of doneness. If meat is boneless or very large, turn it at least once while cooking.

Exotic roasts (moose, venison) cook better in a covered roaster, with water added (for steam), and for a longer period of time. If possible, place on a rack above the water. If you have no meat thermometer, pierce the meat with a skewer. If the juice runs red, it is rare; pink, medium rare. If the juice is no longer red or pink, the meat is well done or overdone, except for pork and poultry.

Liquid Cooking or Stewing. Meat should be cut into small pieces, about 1″ or smaller. Liquid is added to cover, then the meat is simmered until done. Never boil. The temperature for simmering is no higher than 185° F.

When you are rotating foods, avoid cooking vegetables and meat together, if you intend to freeze any part of the meat for future use. You may not want to follow the same rotation the next time you are eating either the vegetable or the meat.

Pot Roast. To pot roast, add about three to four cups boiling liquid (water, milk, tomato juice, vegetable juice, or cube-frozen gravy) to cover bottom of pan.

Many chemically sensitive persons have a reaction when fats are subjected to high temperature. The fats split into glycerol and the glycerol into the toxin Acrolein. For this reason, and because pot roasting means braising or searing the meat at a high heat, the best way to make a pot roast both wholesome and tasty is to use a crock pot.

VEGETABLES

It is said that the ability of a cook can be judged by the quality, quantity, and variety of vegetable dishes he serves. Surely it is a sin to serve vegetables that are overdone, waterlogged, colorless, and tasteless. It is good to use raw vegetables, whenever possible.

To achieve tastier and more nutritious vegetables, observe these points:

Water. Use as little water as possible and save every drop to be used in soup, stews, gelatin for salad, or beverage. The leftover stock can be frozen in small cubes and used as needed.

Cook as Briefly as Possible. Remove from heat and serve at once when just tender; one should just barely be able to pierce with a fork.

Peeling. Peel only when the skin is tough, bitter, or too rough for cleaning well. Vitamins, minerals, and flavor are concentrated directly under the skins of fruits and vegetables. However, mold accumulates very quickly on root vegetables (those in which the edible part grows underground). Therefore, if you are extremely sensitive to mold, you should avoid preparing these vegetables yourself. You may be able to eat them if you have them peeled for you.

Always Refrigerate Vegetables Until Used. Use them as soon as possible. Keep covered. Food value is quickly and easily lost.

Cover. Use cover while cooking as well as when storing to cut down contact with oxygen.

Seasoning. Always season after cooking, before serving.

Avoid Reheating. Cold, cooked vegetables are very good in salads.

The basic methods for cooking vegetables are as follows:

Steam (Waterless Cooking). The best way to cook vegetables is with steam. Preheat a small amount of water in a heavy pan with a tight lid. Use low heat and keep tightly covered. The vegetables should then be placed on a rack above the water level or in a stainless steel steam basket that fits inside a saucepan. Cook until fork tender. Leave the vegetables uncut and unpeeled whenever possible. A chilled vegetable, shredded or grated, and steamed quickly is delicious.

Pressure Cooking. Use directions given by manufacturer. It is necessary to be very precise as to cooking time or the vegetables will be overcooked. Use a minimum of water and bring to a boil before adding vegetables. Cool immediately and serve at once.

Boiling. Spread the vegetables out in a skillet or a heavy pan with a tight lid, and add barely enough boiling water to cover. Turn heat to low so that the liquid is at a simmer (185° F.) and cook until crisp, not mushy, and drain well. Save all liquid.

Simmering in Milk. When cooking vegetables some of the nutrients are lost in the liquid. This happens to a lesser degree if one uses milk rather than water. Preheat the milk and when adding the vegetables stir them well so they are coated. Do not have heat above a simmer or the milk will boil over, scorch, or curdle. A double boiler may be used.

The vegetables may be covered with the milk or ½ cup of water. For a cream sauce, add thickener at least ten minutes before the vegetables are ready. Add thickener to a little cold liquid, blending well, and stir gradually into the hot milk. If the vegetable has a very short cooking time, prepare the cream sauce first.

Double Boiler Steaming. Place a few tablespoons of water in the top of a double boiler, bring to a boil, and add vegetables. Heat, covered, until most of the water has evaporated or the vegetables are heated through. Then place the top over the bottom of the double boiler in which water is boiling. The amount of water should be adequate but it should not touch the bottom of the top pan. Complete cooking until the vegetables are fork-tender.

Baking. This method diminishes vitamin C, and is not recommended for any food high in the vitamin.

Leafy Vegetables. Shred all leafy vegetables before cooking except very young and small leaves (such as spinach or cress). Whirl dry after washing; this helps keep nutrients in the leaf. Add seasoning after cooking.

Stuffing. Larger vegetables can be partly cooked, scooped-out, and filled with chopped, cooked meats, seafood, or fish which has been mixed with the scooped-out part of the vegetable or with an allowed starch. Bake at 350° F. for thirty minutes until tender.

Freezing. The following vegetables can be prepared for cooking (sliced, cubed), dispersed in a single layer on a cookie sheet, and frozen quickly. It is not necessary to blanch them before freezing. As soon as they are frozen, they should be placed in a suitable container and used as needed (for roasts and stews, salads, garnishes, and so forth):

Carrots	Herbs
Celery	Nutmeats
Celery leaves (chopped)	Onion
Chives	Parsnips
Corn (remove from cob)	Peas
Green beans	Rhubarb
Green pepper	Shellbeans
	Squash

Leftovers. Here are suggestions for leftovers: Arrange in individual portions, wrap and freeze. Arrange TV dinner. Wrap and freeze. Use as soon as possible. Use in salad or next rotated meal. Marinate, if desired. Freeze vegetable juice in small cubes. Place in a bag of cellophane or in wide-mouth jars for use in stews and soups. There is too much water loss for use of vegetable juice in salad.

PART IV

MANAGEMENT of Complex Allergies

CHAPTER 17

How to Detect the Problem

MANY PATIENTS have entered Dr. Eloise Kailin's office, almost without hope, unaware of the impact this meeting would have on their future. Dr. Kailin became their lifeline, guiding them back to a healthier life free of many of the substances in their environment that had been responsible for making life almost unbearable. Dr. Kailin spoonfed them every minute detail; what to eat and how to cook it; what to wear and where to buy it; how to build and furnish a new house, and which products to use for cleaning and maintaining it. Because we think no one could say it better than Dr. Kailin, with her permission we are presenting the following material as she wrote it.

Sensitivity to man-made chemicals in our food, air, and water is by no means rare. Pinning down a diagnosis to a specific allergen is unusually difficult, because people who are subject to this chemical sensitivity are likely to react to several different kinds of chemicals.

For this reason, our diagnostic approach is to exclude simultaneously as many chemicals as possible from the entire environment for about seven to ten days and then to return the individual to his normal environment. If the subject improves dramatically while staying away from environmental chemicals and then becomes sick again when he returns to his normal exposures, we go back again to the restricted regime and add different kinds of chemical allergens, one at a time, to see if we can distinguish which are causing trouble.

During the testing period a patient should remain at home. All the following substances, each of which has caused reactions for some patients, should be avoided:

Drugs and Medications. All kinds, whether used as pills or tablets or on the scalp, hair, or body surfaces, and including those used in the mouth, such as mouthwash or toothpaste. Except those specifically permitted by a doctor, no drugs of any kind should be used by a patient during the testing period. Drugs usually contain dyes, flavorings, preservatives, or excipients.

Pesticides. These include insecticides that may be found in pressurized spray cans in the home and insecticides that are normally present in one's everyday food and water supply. It would apply to moth crystals in the closet, to mothproofed shelf paper (even if it is advertised as odorless) permanently mothproofed sweaters, dry cleaning processes that include mothproofing, paint-on pesticides, or paints and varnishes that contain pesticides.

Petro-chemicals. Chemicals derived from petroleum should be excluded from the home as far as possible. These include mineral oils, engine oils, gasoline and gasoline fumes, paint, diesel fumes, and kerosene. Kerosene is usually found as a carrier for the propellants in spray cans, and as a solvent for inks, as in fresh newsprint, ball-point and felt-tipped pens. Kerosene is also used in the manufacture of detergents.

Other petro-chemicals include varsol, paraffin, floor waxes, and utility gas. Fumes from a gas stove or a gas or oil-fired furnace should be avoided. (All things being equal, one would prefer to test in the summer when furnaces are not in use, but it is not always possible to carry out the study at that time.)

Plastics. Particularly troublesome because they are so widely used and because they are often hidden in products that appear safe from the outside. Problems may be caused either by toxic agents added to keep plastics soft or by smaller plastic molecules that break off from the larger plastic polymers. A person may be sensitive to different kinds of these smaller molecules so that one kind of plastic molecule can be tolerated but not another.

Plastic becomes most offensive when heated because more molecules are airborne. Check all appliances, as well as lamps and light sockets for plastic. The covers of ceiling lighting fixtures or diffusing globes over table lights are often plastic. Synthetic fibers used for fabrics, such as polyester, Acrilan, rayon, nylon, and Dacron are made of plastic, as are Teflon-lined cooking utensils, food wrappers such as soft polyethylene food bags, Saran Wrap, and the plastic resin with which food cans are lined.

Other common plastics one might find in the home include combs and brushes, ball-point pens, toys, shower curtains, folding doors, Milium linings, rug pads, and plastic self-stick shelf or decorating paper, such as Contac and Marvalon wall coverings. Electric blankets, heating pads, and even TV sets have plastic-covered wires.

Solvents. These include alcohols, such as rubbing alcohol or ordinary pure ethyl alcohol; fat solvents; xeroxed, dittoed, or other forms of copied material which may contain benzene, ether, acetone, xylene, or toluol. Usually a solvent can be detected by an odor. If it smells, avoid it. Many kitchen cleaners include solvents to remove stubborn fats and oil films.

Turpentine Family. Derives from pine tree resins and includes certain paints and paint solvents as well as the turpentine you smell in Christmas tree needles and cedar-lined closets or blanket chests. A pine scent is often added to household cleaners or animal bedding.

Water. The only water to be used for drinking, for other beverages, and for cooking during the period of the test will be spring water bottled in glass. To purchase such water, consult the yellow pages of your telephone book. We prefer not to trust well water because many wells have been found to be contaminated with detergent, and many contain pesticides. Distilled water can be used in a pinch, but it is not desirable as a substitute for any length of time, because its use depletes the body of useful salts that are present in spring water. Charcoal-filtered water has the same disadvantage as distilled water. Vegetables may be washed in running tap water and given a final rinse in a small pan of spring water before being cooked in spring water.

Miscellaneous. Chlorine, which is found in bleaches such as Clorox and kitchen scouring powders; ammonias, phenols, and creosols, as in Lysol disinfectant; menthol and camphor, as found in Vicks Vaporub and cough medications. Smoke is a potential source of trouble and particularly hard to avoid. This is true of burning fat which produces smoke in the process of quick-frying, as well as the various forms of tobacco and wood smoke. Traffic fumes and smog are generally petro-chemical fumes and must be avoided.

The fungicide Thiram is usually used to manufacture rubber. Anyone sensitive to this fungicide should avoid anything that contains rubber in any form, including rug pads.

By now it should be amply apparent just how difficult it is to avoid all of these everyday exposures all at once. We will consider a practical application of this objective in terms of *additives to the water, to air, and to food.*

Additives to Air Involve Attention to the Following Points: Cook exclusively with electric appliances such as hot plates, electric fry-pans (not Teflon lined) electric broilers, and the like for the rest of the family as well as the affected person. If there is a gas stove in the kitchen, it is most important that the pilot light be turned off before starting the test. Further, the burners are to be wrapped in aluminum foil and sealed with freezer tape so that none of the tar-like deposits in and on the burners will exchange molecules with the air.

Remove from the house—preferably to an outdoor garage or at least to the basement in sealed cans—all substances that smell. This includes paints, solvents, turpentine, all pressurized spray cans, lacquers, kerosene lighter fluid and fire-starting solutions of one sort or another, glues, nail polish and its remover, scented soaps and other cosmetics such as hair spray, deodorants, shoe polish, metal polishes, furniture polish, floor waxes, mops and rags that have been used for oiling or for waxing, detergents, bleaches, ammonia, and any cleaners that have an odor. The cleaners you can use are Bon-Ami, preferably the cake, Rokeach kosher soap, Arm & Hammer washing soda, and pure castile soap.

All pesticides of any kind must be removed from the household. Coffee cans with plastic lids and large galvanized garbage cans make convenient containers for putting away such things as cosmetics, shoe polishes, and felt-tip pens. Anything else you can find that has a distinct odor to it, particularly if it is in one of the families of chemicals outlined earlier, should be similarly eliminated.

If there are oil-sprayed or hexachlorophene-treated filters in either heating or cooling equipment, these should be replaced with clean metal mesh filters which may be sprayed with olive oil for better adhesiveness of dust particles. It is almost impossible to buy air-conditioner filters that have not been treated with the chlorinated hydrocarbon hexachlorophene; even the untreated filters contain a resin coating on the glass fibers.

Bedroom. Insofar as possible, the bedroom of the person undergoing this study should be free from soft plastic containers such as garment bags. If the person has a dust allergy, and there is a soft plastic cover on the mattress and springs, usually the best compromise is to use extra-heavy toweling or a blanket between the bottom sheet and the plastic casing. Occasionally it is necessary to use a canvas army cot and dispense with the mattress and its plastic cover.

In any event, the pillow must not be rubber or plastic foam or of a plastic, fiber-filled type such as Dacron, Dynel, polyester, poly-foam or polyurethane. While he is being tested for chemical sensitivity, a person sensitive to dust should use a folded, cotton sheet-blanket for a pillow.

We are usually not concerned with hard plastics, such as Formica or the old hard Bakelite. Such plastics would only be a problem if heated to a fairly high degree. Soft plastics, particularly the new ones that still have an odor about them, frequently cause quite a bit of trouble. Electric blankets are absolutely out because the heating of their plastic-coated wires releases a rather severe plastic-fume load, even though it does not carry much of an odor.

Clothing. Clothing is a major problem during the testing period. The clothing must be free both of detergent residue from the laundry and from plastic fiber content. It also must be free from the plastic finishes that render most of our modern clothing drip-dry, crease-resistant, or stain-resistant. In purchasing cotton fabrics, a quick practical test may be made by carrying a small bottle of water and putting a drop on the fabric of new clothing. If the drop stays bubbled-up on the surface, do not buy the item. The aim is to find untreated clothing, from underwear on out, made of natural fibers, such as cotton, silk, wool, or linen. Rayon should not be used during this testing period. Cotton-knit material which is not bonded is desirable, and the kind of knit shirts found in sporting departments are frequently satisfactory. Older clothing and blankets which are pesticide free are cherished when we find we have to live with this kind of problem. Women's stockings should be cotton lisle or real silk, and may be obtained in limited colors in major department stores. Often men must be content with cotton socks that contain a small amount of nylon reinforcement around the toe. Blue jeans and chinos or painters' pants for men, or cotton-cord summer clothing, can sometimes be used during this testing period, although it gets harder every year to find untreated materials. Women should use garter belts rather than plastic stretch, Lycra, or rubber girdles or wear pants and cotton socks. There should be a minimum amount of plastic or rubber in undergarments. None of these clothes should be worn with new sizing or fillers in them. Before the study begins, each article should be laundered in pure unperfumed soap, like Rokeach kosher soap, and/or baking soda, and/or Arm & Hammer washing soda, or borax.

Personal Care. A bath and a shampoo are essential before the study starts to remove any traces of cosmetics or detergents from hair, scalp, and skin. Of course soap is limited to pure unperfumed soap. Neither hair sprays nor cosmetics may be used by women, and men must forego shaving soaps and lotions. Electric razors are perfectly acceptable.

Ice water may be used as an astringent. No mouth washes may be used during the testing period, and the teeth may be brushed only with salt and soda. If douches or enemas are desired during the testing period, spring water should be used. Contraceptives, if needed during the testing period, should be limited to rubber or sheath-skin condoms, without the use of the usual contraceptive jelly. This is risky, and abstention is suggested.

Smoke. The smoking of tobacco *by anyone in the house* during the testing period is completely prohibited, and it will not be possible for the person undergoing the test to go to work or to school unless it can be assured that these environments will be free of smoke, cosmetics, fumes, perfumes, oils, floor waxes, and other airborne substances of the kinds described. It will also be necessary to avoid trips into stores and parking lots where smoke or smog might be encountered. Quite often automobiles will have a strong odor of gasoline or from plastics and these should be avoided.

Food. Finding additive-free foods means that one must find foods that have been grown without the use of weed killers or pesticides, and that these foods have been transported and handled in such a manner that they are not contaminated by further spraying, plastic food wrappers, the addition of preservatives, dyes, or so-called freshening agents.

If food, otherwise properly handled, has been kept in a plastic container but not heat-sealed, it is possible to remove the food from its plastic container and let it air for about three days. The plastic factor will evaporate so that the food can then be used.

However, if food has been heat-sealed in plastic as is often the case with meats, and is always the case with foods in tin cans, it contains such a large number of the smaller plastic molecules that we cannot rely on airing it to free it from plastic contamination. Crisp cellophane wrappers appear to be less contaminated than the soft polyethylene ones.

(In the Washington, D.C., area, the Kennedy Natural Food Center, 1051 West Broad Street, Falls Church, Virginia, Tel. (703) 533-8484, makes a specialty of gathering additive-free food. In other areas, have your local health food store manager contact James Kennedy, who has agreed to discuss methods of helping your local store meet your needs.)

There are a few food items in your ordinary market that are relatively free from chemical contamination. These include dry, powdered skim milk, and you may use frozen okra, frozen cooked squash, and frozen lima beans, if you limit your choice to those in waxed cartons. You may use ordinary tomato juice—in glass—but not a cocktail mix. Frozen Alaska King crab or frozen South African lobster tails, provided these have not been heat-sealed in plastic, are acceptable, as are parsley, melon, and Jerusalem artichokes.

If you are able to get fish that has been frozen and packed in Iceland, this is usually tolerated well. Bananas from any source are acceptable if they have not been treated with ethylene gas to ripen them. Naturally ripened bananas can be distinguished by the presence of many fine, little, brown speckled spots as opposed to large brown blazes caused by the gas.

Food Preparation. When you have made your food purchases you must then store, prepare, and cook them. You should acquire a good thick roll of cellophane or parchment paper to be used instead of Saran Wrap or waxed paper. Do not cook in any aluminum cooking utensil since heated aluminum, for some reason not yet fathomed, is sometimes a problem. Preferably use Corningware, Pyrex, enamel, stainless steel, or cast-iron cooking utensils. Salt is limited to sea salt or chemically pure sodium chloride. Do not allow foods to char or cooking fats to smoke. Cook slowly or cook with water. Do not fry because of the smoke that results. Steaming is an excellent way to cook vegetables as it saves vitamins and flavor.

Store leftovers in glass, china, pottery, or similar containers, but not in plastics. Atlas, Ball, or Triomphe freezer jars (be sure the lids have no plastic), or Pyrex refrigerator dishes are convenient for leftovers. Wash dishes with tap water and a pure unperfumed soap like Rokeach's Kosher soap. Dry with detergent-free cloth towels (bleach in paper towels may cause trouble). Keep all special foods tightly covered in the refrigerator except those being aired to remove plastic fumes. Removal of odors in the refrigerator, and airing of foods once wrapped in plastic, can be facilitated by placing a bag of activated coconut charcoal in the refrigerator.

CHECK LIST AND TIMETABLE

First, determine what nonperishable purchases will be necessary: clothing, cooking equipment, cleaners, water, staple foods.

Second, schedule a conference with the doctor.

Third, arrange to have the gas stove turned off and arrange for absence from school or work.

Fourth, clear the house of solvents, cosmetics, pesticides and plastics.

Fifth and last, obtain perishable foods.

Keep close notes of what you eat and how you feel. Schedule a conference with the doctor toward the end of your additive-free period, and be sure to remain on the special restrictions. The conference is very important because if you show a great deal of improvement, the doctor may elect to allow you your normal exposures in separate categories rather than allow all of them at once. This would save time in the long run, if there is strong reason to believe you have chemical intolerances.

You should bear in mind that true freedom is freedom to choose knowledgeably. Illness from unknown causes destroys your freedom. The more closely the causes of illness can be pinpointed, the greater your freedom. Therefore, after your testing period has been completed and you are well into your program, go on a binge if you feel restrictions hem you in—but you should also be free to feel well.

TEST ADDITIONS

When you are chemically free, this is how to test for individual classes of substances—*one at a time.* Allow at least two to three days between tests of different categories.

Do you have trouble from any of these?

Tap Water. Use in place of spring water.

Insecticides. Use market fruits, green vegetables in place of organic foods (after having restricted your diet to organic foods for at least one week).

Food Dyes. Test red, yellow, green, blue, one drop of each by mouth on successive days.

Butter. One teaspoon by mouth first day, 1 tablespoon on second and third day.

Jello. One kind each day, 1 tablespoon serving. Do not test if your dye tests are positive.

Plastics. Food: put tolerated oil into flexible plastic food container twenty-four to forty-eight hours. Immerse soft plastic food bag in it. Add 1 tablespoon of that oil to salad. (Do not heat the oil before testing plastic factor.) Clothing: Orlon, nylon, Dacron. Wear next to skin overnight and wear synthetics the next day.

Use of Gas Stove. Sit in kitchen with oven lit for two hours. If no ill effects, eat potato or other food baked in oven.

Clorox. One tablespoon in 1 cup water: use ½ teaspoon of this mixture on blotter, four feet away, fifteen to twenty minutes' exposure.

Ammonia. One tablespoon in 1 cup water: use ½ teaspoon of this mixture on blotter, four feet away, fifteen to twenty minutes' exposure.

Moth Balls (paradichlorobenzene). One half teaspoon four to six feet away in small room, fifteen to twenty minutes.

Use of Detergents. Rinse out face cloth in Tide or All. Hold near face for fifteen minutes.

Rubber Foam or Plastic Foam. Smell a piece for twenty to thirty minutes. If no ill effects, use a pillow of foam overnight.

Fairprene (synthetic rubber dust-proofing material for mattress casings). Test as a pillow case.

Fresh Newsprint. Hold freshly printed newspaper six to seven inches from nose ten to fifteen minutes.

Lipstick. Test individual colors on separate days.

Deodorant. Test underarm.

Aspirin. Test corn-free (if required) as individually instructed only if aspirin sensitivity is suspected; reaction can be violent.

Acetone (nail polish remover). Few drops on blotter two feet away for twenty minutes' exposure.

Shellac. Few drops on blotter two feet away for twenty minutes' exposure.

Turpentine. Few drops on blotter two feet away for twenty minutes' exposure.

Kerosene. Few drops on blotter two feet away for twenty minutes' exposure.

Gasoline. Stand near gas station pump for five to ten minutes' exposure.

Car Exhaust Fumes. Stand near bus stop for five to ten minutes' exposure.

CHAPTER 18

How to Begin a Toxic-Free Life

O NCE CHEMICAL sensitivities have been diagnosed, what are the first steps to be taken? There will be many changes to make if you wish to eliminate the things that make you ill.

First, make a list of the various functions of your daily life and the objects that you must use in connection with them.

You will be surprised at how many important things you must consider, such as newspapers, telephone, bedding, and heat. Many chapters of this book will give you tips on what to do about the products to which you are sensitive. Make a note beside each item on your list of what you plan to do to clear your environment. You may never reach the ultimate goal of solving all your problems, but you can take giant steps toward achieving a relatively toxic-free existence.

Some of the following material repeats what appears elsewhere, but the intention here is to help you decide the order of importance for your attention and to present it in a format that is easy to use.

The three priorities are the bedroom, clothing, and food:

BEDROOM

Bed and Bedding. The ideal situation is to use the smallest bedroom in the house. Remove everything from the closet, and strip the bedroom except for a bed, a table, a clock, a lamp, and anything considered a necessity such as a telephone or small, old radio made of wood or metal. The bed should have an untreated cotton mattress. Test barrier cloth (see p. 230) and, if you can tolerate it, order a zippered mattress cover made of this fabric. Bedding and curtains should be made of untreated cotton which has been washed in pure soap, washing soda, baking soda, and/or borax.

If you are mildly allergic you may think this doesn't apply to you. However, people often blame the wrong things for their problems. For example, although Judy, a young girl who knew she was allergic to dust, made every effort to keep her bedroom dust-free, the mattress always retained a residual amount of dust. She suffered nightly from a stuffy nose and blamed it on her mattress. However, when she slept at a friend's home she had no difficulty. She discovered that her friend did not use detergent in her laundry. When Judy discontinued using detergent, her difficulty cleared up.

Bookcases. Bookcases and desks should be avoided. There should be no paper or books in closets, drawers, or anywhere in the room. Especially in the beginning, you need as much as eight hours daily in a pure environment. The purer it is, the faster the recovery. If there is ample room in the house, it is wise to clear out another room such as a sunroom or family room. Of course, the kitchen should be as clear as possible. The doors to all rooms should be closed.

Carpeting. Avoid carpeting. If rugs are used, they should be cotton scatter rugs that can be easily and frequently washed. Scatter rugs should not be backed with plastic, rubber, or glue substances. They cannot be nonskid, so one must walk carefully. Rugs can be anchored by the furniture.

Closets. When the bedroom and closet cannot be completely stripped, the contents should be limited to 100 percent untreated cotton. In the closet, there should be no shoes, purses, clothes that have been dry-cleaned, paper, or plastic (which includes any synthetic fabric such as nylon, Acrilan, Dacron, rayon, fiber-glass material, and drip-dry or permanent press clothes).

Beware of "nonallergenic" Dynel pillows, imitation leather products, furniture polishes, and floor waxes. Formica furniture usually is no problem, however.

When irritants must be kept in the closet, seal the bottom of the closet door with material covered with heavy-duty aluminum, thus closing off fumes.

Dresser. If there is a dresser in the bedroom, it should be checked as carefully as the closet. It should be free of perfumes and sachet odors. Do not store any kind of cosmetics, plastic jewelry, sprays of any kind, deodorant, any scented products, or any plastic accessories in a dresser. Other items to be avoided are plastic lamps with plastic sockets, shades, clocks, picture frames, any paper or cardboard articles.

Old dressers should be checked to see that they do not contain residues of perfumes and other toxic substances that have been stored in them. New dressers should be checked. Unfortunately most new dressers are made with treated wood and/or are treated for insecticides and/or are varnished.

Table. A safe kind of bedroom table is made of wrought iron with a glass top.

Telephone. Very sensitive persons who must have a phone in the bedroom should ask the telephone company for an old metal telephone with cloth wires.

Many persons are bothered by new wire. If you pester the officials often enough and long enough, the telephone company may find an old-fashioned, metal telephone with cloth-bound wire. Ask to speak to the general manager, but settle for a high-ranking supervisor. Tell them that other branches have found metal phones for patients, so you know it is possible. Warn the officials in advance not to clean the phones. (one phone when found was cleaned with an oil-based cleaner and could never be used.)

Most people don't know that telephones contain a wad of cotton impregnated with fungicide.[1] One woman we know of could not be in the same room with a telephone until this wad of cotton was found and removed. The wad is often tucked down in the "throat of the handset and may require tweezers or the point of a knife to fish it out. This remedy has brought comfort overnight to several chemically sensitive individuals who were bothered by their phone.

Use a phone with a jack. When the phone is not in use, remove it from the bedroom.

Heat. As hot-air heat, even if it is electric, can cause trouble because of oils in the fan and for other reasons, it should be turned off in the bedroom. Seal off the vent with a couple of layers of aluminum foil taped with freezer paper tape. If heat is needed, you should buy an International Hot Water Unit.[2] This unit can be ordered directly from the company, with the request that it be stripped of plastic and paint. Because the company is accustomed to dealing with patients with sensitivities, they will be familiar with your request.

If possible, the room should be kept very warm while you are away from it so that the unit can be turned off while you are there. Some highly sensitive people react even to this kind of unit. A room with a sunny exposure can be of great help. However, it is more important to take a room where the windows face away from the street so that the patient is exposed to the least amount of traffic fumes.

CLOTHING

Cleaning Clothes. After the testing period is over, you can determine how careful you have to be with cleaning procedures. Until then, observe the greatest precautions in choosing the best ways to wash clothes. During the testing period it is best not to have clothes dry-cleaned. To clean the family's clothes, send them to a dry cleaner who will use naphtha, which is believed to be the least offensive commercial product. The clothes must then be aired thoroughly before the patient can be exposed to them.

Untreated Cotton. As with everything else, clothing in the beginning should be very simple; experimenting with a variety of fabrics can come later. At first 100 percent pure cotton should be used. Because dyes can be a problem for some people, strong dyes should be avoided. Pastel colors and off-whites are more easily tolerated than the darker dyes.

FOOD

Rotation. The first priority is avoidance of foods to which you are allergic. Rotation of foods is recommended (see Chapter 8).

Sources. Once the diet is planned, the next step is to learn the sources of food relatively free of contaminants (preservatives, insecticides, and additives). Even if your health food store does not carry organic produce or other organic products, they can usually refer you to any local source. Otherwise, the Kennedy Natural Food Store has agreed to supply the information if you get in touch with them. Or if you wish they will ship foods to you. Send for their catalog.[3] Rodale Press publishes sources of organic foods.

Preparation. Whenever possible, foods should be eaten uncooked.

Cooking and Eating Utensils. Food should be prepared with pots, pans, dishes, and silverware that are not made of plastic, Teflon, or aluminum. It may also be necessary to use the same precaution when food is being cooked for other people in the house. The danger comes from the odors of the heated aluminum and/or plastic.

Cooking Odors. A precaution about food prepared for the rest of the family: some highly sensitive persons cannot tolerate even the odor of foods to which they are allergic. Such persons should keep the kitchen as well ventilated as possible and leave the kitchen frequently, returning only when necessary for the preparation of the food. Whenever a member of your family is cooking, even though it's not for you, he must know what precautions are necessary for your special needs.

CHAPTER 19

Tips for the Beginner

BEFORE YOU do anything else, stop! Don't panic. Relax. It wouldn't surprise us at all if you feel overwhelmed. In the beginning, most people do.

Take our word for it, it is possible to achieve a normal life style.

To aid you in this initial adjustment, we have prepared, in capsule form, the facts that most acutely sensitive persons need to know: some Do's and Don'ts.

First, we strongly advise that you do your testing for allergies and sensitivities under the supervision of a clinical ecologist. (If you need the name of one in your area, get in touch with Dr. Robert Collier, the secretary of the Society for Clinical Ecology.[1] After completion of testing, you may find that some of these tips do not apply to you. Until then, it is important that you do not take chances, but wait until your particular sensitivites are established by the doctor.

Avoid Snap Decisions. Do not make any hasty major decisions without first consulting your doctor or a knowledgeable person. When buying a home, if possible stay for several days in the new place before signing on the dotted line, or rent before buying. For example, when one patient discovered she was allergic to gas and oil, she signed a lease in an all-electric building. Unfortunately, once a week, in that building, an exterminator sprayed chemicals which were worse for the patient than gas and oil.

Reading Box. If you are sensitive to these printed pages, we recommend that you buy an inexpensive picture frame with glass and read under the glass. To avoid fumes that accumulate under the glass, some patients build or buy a reading box.

If cost is no object, the more practical box is one which can be purchased from Human Ecology Equipment Design and Fabrication Co. at 413 Betty Jo Lane, Garland, Texas 75042. Since sensitivity extends to different woods and even metals, the company carries a variety to let you choose one you can tolerate. The professionally made box is designed so that when your hands are inside the box, they are covered with pure cotton gloves made of barrier cloth.

For an additional cost, a stand is available that adjusts to different heights so that the box can be tilted for comfortable reading angles.

You can make your own reading box. The following instructions are those of Peter Sulzer, a friend who made two reading boxes as samples for us:

How to Make Your Own Box. "The reading box consists of a shallow glass-covered aluminum box that permits the reader to be protected from the volatile components of a book while he reads. The pages are turned by means of a slender rod that is inserted through a slot along the front side of the box.

"I made one from a Bud Radio Co. AC-420 unpainted aluminum chassis base which can be purchased from a radio parts store. This base is 13″ by 17″ by 3″ deep, which is large enough for most books.

"Use a piece of window glass, single strength, 13″ by 17″, as a cover. The sharp edges of the glass should be dulled with sandpaper.

"Fasten the glass to the base with steel angles that are positioned to come up the sides of the chassis base and over the glass (for about 1″), so that the glass will not fall off. Use these angles along only three sides of the glass, so that the reader can slide the glass of the open face of the chassis to permit insertion or removal of the book. On this open face of the chassis (17″ by 3″), cut a slot about ¼″ wide and 15″ long. This slot should be positioned about 1″ down from the open face of the base. Cut the slot by drilling three ¼″ holes at each end and then joining the holes with a hacksaw, finishing with a file. The hacksaw blade has to be turned 90° from its normal position in the hacksaw frame.

"Make the rod from a 12″ piece of ³⁄₁₆″ dowel, suitably pointed at one end.

"I recommend a small bag of activated charcoal to be placed inside the box to help absorb the fumes.

"To read, place the open book inside box, replace the glass. Through the open slot at the front, slide the pointed rod separating the top page of the book from the rest of the book, then turn the page. With a little practice, it becomes easier."

Larger boxes can be made to accommodate larger books.

If you cannot tolerate even the slight exposure of the fumes escaping from the reading box, and have no one to read to you, ask your doctor to write to the National Foundation for the Blind; you will be qualified for reader volunteers.

TIPS TO AVOID PLASTICS

Bakelite. Many products used daily are not necessarily recognized as plastics. Bakelite is one example. Bakelite handles on pots and pans should not be exposed unnecessarily to heat. Phenol and formaldehyde are very important components of Bakelite, emitting fumes at the slightest heat. Only a few patients are bothered by the hard Bakelite in the telephone.

Ball-point Pens. Ink solvent is the problem here. Felt-tip and magic-marker pens are even worse. Use pencil whenever possible, or use a metal ball-point pen. We find Cross least offensive.

Combs, Plastic. Aluminum combs are available at natural food stores and some drugstores. Also, inquire about wooden combs. Ivory, though expensive, is ideal. Tortoise shell is also fine.

Contact Lens. Contact lenses are plastic.

Containers. Avoid plastic, soft or hard, even Tupperware. The best containers are glass Mason jars with wide-mouth tops of enamel and red rubber.

Cutlery. Avoid plastic-handled knives, spoons, and forks. Use stainless steel.

Dentures. Avoid plastic dentures. Tell your dentist that enamel dentures, though expensive, can be obtained from York Dental Supply in New York City.

Dishes and Cooking Utensils. Avoid plastic tablewear. Inexpensive enameled pots are usable only until chipped. Since they chip so easily, they become expensive. Corningware (dishes and pots) and Pyrex or Fire-King are practical choices. An excellent, though expensive, choice is Descoware, made of cast iron coated with baked-on enamel.

Doors. Avoid plastic doors.

Dress Shields. Dress shields and shoulder pads in clothing have a plastic base. Make your own with barrier cloth.

Eyeglasses. Avoid plastic frames and lenses, including aluminum frames that are plastic-coated. Avoid using plastic close to your eyes, ears, and nose as in plastic eyeglasses (use aluminum or frameless with glass lenses). Gold nosepieces can be obtained if you are sensitive even to hard plastic. Use leather eyeglass cases.

Hair Brushes. Use natural-bristle wooden-handled hairbrushes, available at natural food centers and most department stores.

Lamps. Check lamps and sockets for plastic. Heated plastic is most offensive. Ceiling-light covers or diffusing globes over table lights are often plastic.

Rug Pads. We know of no safe rug pad. Best do without. Instead, anchor rugs by strategically placing heavy furniture at the corners of the rugs. We do know that the newer rug pads are becoming more and more toxic.

Shelf Paper. Added pesticides often increase the toxicity of the plastic of self-stick decorating paper or shelf paper. Instead, use aluminum foil or aluminum wallpaper.

Shower Curtains. During testing period, use a homemade shower curtain of terrycloth, barrier cloth, or a linen tablecloth. Throw over top of bar and place safety pins two or three inches apart. Get rid of that plastic shower curtain.

Stationery. Many kinds of paper are plastic-coated. Smell paper before buying it.

Teflon. Avoid anything Teflon-coated, including electric irons. Use distilled water in the iron, and spring water if clothes must be sprinkled. Be sure the ironing board cover and pad are pure cotton (not treated with asbestos or Teflon).

Avoid Teflon and other plastic-coated cookware. If you are buying new pans, Pyrex and Corningware are most satisfactory except for frying, for which enamel-coated cast iron or iron skillets are suggested. Inexpensive safe pots are Columbian enamel (but there is the danger of chipping). Avoid aluminum pots, too.

Traverse Rods. Traverse rods are usually plastic. Round wooden or metal decorator rods should be used.

Wallets. Use leather wallets without the plastic credit card and picture compartments.

Wrapping. Avoid plastic wrapping for food as well as clothes bags, furniture covers, and small appliance covers. Remove foods from plastic containers, air for three or four days, and repackage in glass jars or cellophane.[2]

MISCELLANEOUS TIPS

Adhesive. Johnson & Johnson adhesive is much less odorous than Parke-Davis or Bauer and Black.

Air Freshener. Pomanders give out a delightful fragrance that freshens the air for months. Stick cloves into an orange, as many cloves as you can. Hang in cotton tulle netting. Peppermint sprigs in the garbage can and around the house help odors disappear naturally.

Anesthetics. Most likely to succeed: Pentothal, first choice, if there is no barbiturate sensitivity. Demerol, codeine (hypotabs or injection). Halothane, if inhaled gas anesthetic is required.

Asbestos. Avoid excessive use of asbestos, which can be found in vinyl flooring, wallpapers, insulation, Contac paper, stove mitts, and pot holders, as well as wiring.

Bath Water. A few crystals of sodium thiosulfate changes chlorine in water to chloride; it may be helpful to chlorine-sensitive persons for bathing only—not to be used internally.

Christmas Trees. These can contribute to indoor pollution. We know an artist who had to stop using oil paints because he developed hives every time he used turpentine. He could never understand why he always suffered from hives during the Christmas holiday. Once he learned that turpentine is derived from pine tree resin and stopped buying Christmas trees, he was able to enjoy a Christmas without hives.

Some sensitive people can tolerate a southern hemisphere evergreen, the Norfolk Island Pine. Available at nurseries and some florists, these make beautiful year-around potted plants, which can be decorated for Christmas. Other people have created their own trees of papier-mâché using coat hangers or umbrella stands.

Cooking. Avoid aluminum when cooking; aluminum is toxic when heated, the heavy aluminum as much so as the less expensive aluminum pans. Use stainless steel baking tins and cooking tools.[3]

Cleaning Tip. Smooth creamy peanut butter can remove asphalt and tar from a child's skin and hair. Rub it in well and soon the sticky substances will loosen.

Clothing. Cape: If it is necessary to have an outdoor garment other than a coat, a convenient solution is a cape of heavy wide-wale corduroy lined with the same material, making it reversible (for warmth as well as for appearance).

Cotton Handkerchiefs. Keep a clean one wrapped in foil in your pocket and use it to protect nose when noxious fumes cannot be avoided. This is frequently better than charcoal filters, for the latter are difficult for some to tolerate.

Don't throw away old clothes: After your acute stage is over, you may find that you can tolerate some old synthetics but not new ones. Also, certain synthetics lose some of their toxicity in time. In the beginning, stick to cotton clothes marked 100 percent cotton or all-cotton. Be sure they are untreated. Do not use drip-dry or soil-release fabrics as there are plastic coatings on the cotton fibers.

Morning Robe. If you have trouble finding one, use a terry-cloth robe marked 100 percent cotton. Challis (cotton and wool) makes a beautiful robe and it is washable.

Slippers. Until you can find 100 percent leather morning slippers, use 100 percent cotton ankle socks.

Cloths. Unbleached flour sacks from Sears Roebuck and Montgomery Ward can be used for utility cloths.

Corningware. Although Corningware is usually good, the automatic skillet has a bad odor when new. Check all electrical units in the store before buying anything.

Cosmetics. Avoid cosmetics with petroleum base and/or perfume. Be careful of cosmetics on other persons. Stay upwind and keep your distance. Present your loved one with the kind you can tolerate.

Detergents. Avoid detergents for washing dishes and clothes. Automatic dishwashers should not be used because of plastic parts and the need for detergent. When dishes are drying, these fumes are carried through the house.

Diapers. Avoid the use of disposable diapers.

Eating Tips. Avoid eating when in pain, feverish, or in mental and physical discomfort. Do not drink with meals and avoid ice-cold or too-hot drinks.

Erasers. The fine side of an emery board can be used to erase type and ball-point pen markings.

Food and Preparation. All foods in health stores are not organic. Look for labels marked: "Prepared without preservatives or additives," "Made of foods grown without chemicals."

Not all bottled water is pure spring water. Be sure your water is marked with both words, "Spring Water." Be sure the water is bottled in glass, not plastic. Final rinse of all foods must be with spring water.

Cook with electricity only. If you do not have an electric stove, buy a portable oven and a "metal plate" electric burner.

Food Storage. Moisture-proof cellophane bags may be ordered from Nuvita Foods.[4] They come with ties, are especially good to use in freezing, and food stored in them is tolerated well by some sensitive people. Sizes from one to ten pounds. Size 2 fits nicely in Dine-out cartons which then may be stacked in the freezer. Size 4 fits well in E-Z freezer containers with aluminum-coated lids. These containers should not come in direct contact with food.

Gasoline. Use unleaded gasoline. Be sure to tell the attendant to stop at the first click of the automatic pump. (Additional pumping by hand results in spillage, wastes gas and causes toxic fumes.)

Glue. Glue-Bird glue is nontoxic and recommended for heavier gluing when Elmer's glue, which is also nontoxic, is not strong enough.

Hexachlorophene. Beware of hexachlorophene in soap and furnace filters. This is a chlorinated hydrocarbon like DDT.

Kitchen Utensils. Ice cube trays: Replace plastic liners with all-metal trays; do be careful to wash new metal trays with hot soapy water until sprayed-on "no-stick" finish is removed.

Vacuum Bottles. Stainless steel vacuum bottles can be purchased at hunting stores.

Lanolin. Lanolin marked pure must be bought with discrimination. If you are not sure of its safety, make it yourself. Toilet Lanolin is not pure lanolin.

Light Bulbs. Avoid "Perma-lite" long life light bulbs which are sold via telephone by handicapped workers. Apparently some form of plastic is used in giving the bulbs their extra life. (One patient had an instant and severe plastic reaction from using such a bulb.)

Lubrication. One patient finds she can tolerate graphite for lubricating her sewing machine and zippers. Check first with your repairman.

Mothproofing. Dr. Eloise Kailin was quoted in a newspaper column nationally distributed by the Los Angeles Times syndicate on the perils of using the chemical dieldrin in mothproofing of rugs. "I have established that dieldrin does not stay in the mothproofed rug," Dr. Kailin says in the article. "With wear, particles of the rug break off and become ordinary house dust that people breathe. When it passes over heated surfaces, it generates other toxic gases. With our chronic exposure to hard pesticides and hundreds of mildly toxic chemicals, our ability to tolerate further exposures is breaking down."

Oil. For relatively odor-free automobile oil use RPM or Quaker State.

Paper. Do not use colored or perfumed household papers of any kind. The paper dissolves but the dyes remain, polluting soil and water and contaminating your indoor environment. Some gynecologists say that perfume in tissue, sanitary pads, and tampons and feminine deodorants are dangerous, often causing vaginitis.

Paper Towels. Avoid using paper towels, even white, unperfumed towels, to drain food and dry dishes; they are treated with bleaches and contain starch.

Purifiers. If indoor air becomes polluted, causing you trouble, check with your allergist about using charcoal bags or charcoal room air purifiers.

Shampoos. Try Jheri Redding Milk 'n Honee or Amino Pon; neither contain perfume and both seem to help dandruff. When there's no time for a regular shampoo, dust arrowroot or corn starch on your hair, brush it out; excess oil and dirt will be absorbed and your hair will emerge fluffy.

Soap. Rokeach kosher soap (available at supermarkets and small stores catering to a Jewish clientele) is a pure coconut oil soap good for dishes, pots and pans, and household cleaning.[5]

Warning: Read labels very carefully. Sometimes new products are packaged so that they closely resemble others but do not have the same degree of purity, or may be a different product by the same company. For example, one woman recently bought what she thought was the Arm & Hammer borax she used regularly. She took it home and discovered it was a new detergent by the same company. A short time ago a doctor sent us a label that looked identical to the wrapper found on the "99$\frac{44}{100}$ percent pure" Ivory soap bar. However, on close examination, the label indicated it was a detergent complexion bar.

CHAPTER 20

Making Life Easier

UNFORTUNATELY, in the beginning, at the time that your reactions are most severe, and it is difficult to manage simple shopping, you will have to make major changes in clothing, cooking utensils, and furnishings. To make your adjustment easier, this chapter outlines some of the methods that have proved most helpful.

The telephone and forthrightness are your two best tools. You will be surprised at how much cooperation you will receive if you explain briefly that you are allergic to many things in a store, and a lengthy stay there would make you ill. Try to find a department store where usually you can deal with the same person. You will get better attention if you deal with a supervisor.

Sears's catalog department is frequently an excellent source. Call the manager, explain your problem, and arrange to work with the same individual each time. (At Sears salespersons are not permitted to divulge their names, but they can give you their catalog code number.) If you explain your problem, they will even look through the catalog for you for items you need and will call you back. Do not leave anything up to their judgment. Since you will usually get only what you ask for, be sure to outline every detail of the service you need.

Whenever possible, have things delivered. If you must pick up a package, find out the exact charge and tell the salesperson you will have a check or the exact amount of money ready. Ask her to have the bill completed. If using a charge plate, ask the salesperson to have the slip completely filled out with items and cost, so you will have to wait only for the plate to be stamped and your signature added.

Learn the name or number of the salesperson so you will know whom to ask for. Make an appointment with the salesperson for the time you will be there so she will be expecting you. If you are going to a place where you have to draw a check and wait your turn (at Sears the pickup clerk is different from the order clerk), arrange with the supervisor to have someone there waiting to take you out of turn.

If you tell the supervisor of your store that this arrangement is available at other Sears stores, it might convince him to cooperate in a similar manner.

Cotton Items. In the beginning, it is better to stick to cotton because it is the easiest to buy by phone and easy to wash. (Dry-cleaning can be a problem.) On the phone explain the following to the salesperson: The item must be marked 100 percent cotton or all cotton, and it must be untreated.

Be considerate. Ask the salesperson to call you back when she has no other customer in the store. Ask her to test the material by placing a drop of water on it. If the cotton absorbs the water immediately, it may be safe. It is unsafe if the water forms beads and remains on top. This applies only to cotton—100 percent cotton.

When possible, buy in quantity with the understanding that you will wash and test one garment and return the others if something irritates you, such as the dyes. Explain that you want to buy in quantity because very often by the time you have tested articles they are no longer available, and it is so difficult to find things. Charge whenever possible, and be sure the things are returnable. When shopping by phone, try to get solid colors. Stick to light colors; avoid dark colors because dark dyes are the most offensive. You cannot test things in advance for catalog buying at Sears, but they are very good about returns.

Using this method you can buy underwear, pajamas, double-knit blouses, shorts and slacks, socks, tablecloths, towels, sheets, pillow cases, and yardgoods. Wash before using. Try to avoid buying dresses, robes, and suits. You are better off having them made because some synthetics are used for facing and decorations.

Hairdresser. To most allergic people a beauty shop is now a naughty word. In Chapter 28 you will find suggestions of substitutes for cosmetics, but the real problem solver is a hairdresser's willingness to come to your home. Call the nearest beauty parlor first. For a price, you can usually find someone. The main expense comes from the distance the beautician has to travel. There are a few ways to find a beautician who lives close by.

Advertise for a beautician or former beautician who would like to pick up extra money helping a neighbor who is allergic to beauty shops. Put up notices in neighborhood stores, apartment buildings, recreational centers, churches. To help you find someone, ask clergymen, friends, relatives, teachers, clerks.

Housewares. Telephone shopping for pots and pans is comparatively easy. You may, however, have to contact the buyer of the department to make certain that gadgets and cookie and cake tins are free of aluminum, Teflon, or any other plastic.

Shoes. These present a definite problem if you are sensitive to the man-made material of the innersole and the inner lining. Call various stores in advance to ask if they handle brands made completely with leather (like Amalfi). In order to secure fast service from the clerk, tell him your size and ask him to have the shoes out for you to try on. While you wait on the phone (or he can call you back), ask him to check the inside of the soles and the bottom to make sure that in no place does it say man-made material. If you do not tell him where to look and what to look for, you may find that not one pair he has set aside is really all leather.

CHAPTER 21

First Aid and First Aid Supplies: Medical Hints

MORE THAN any other chapter, this one is geared to those who are sensitive to chemicals in general and to drugs specifically. However, even for those of you who are interested only in prevention, there is a great deal that you can learn from this chapter.

If you are trying to be cautious and trying to avoid artificial colors, artificial flavors, and preservatives, it is important for you to note how difficult it is for the clinical ecologist to find medicine, drugs, and vitamins for his patients who cannot tolerate these additives.

You will discover as you read this chapter that there are many common sense treatments that can be used in lieu of some of the products found unsatisfactory for those who are so sensitive.

Medic Alert. The first recommendation is to request a consultation period with your physician to prepare a form for Medic Alert. The dollars invested for a Medic Alert bracelet are well spent. The fee also includes a permanent record at Turlock, California, so that in an emergency, any doctor, anywhere, will be in a position to prescribe treatment with minimum danger of prescribing something to which you are allergic.

On the back of the bracelet is your assigned number, a brief outline of your problem, and a telephone number in Turlock, California, which can be called collect by any doctor who must give you emergency medical treatment.

Keep a copy of the check list so that you too will be prepared. Ask the doctor to recommend a list of drugs for surgery, dental care, eye care, most likely to be tolerated by you, including an antibiotic, anesthesia, pain reliever, local antiseptic, and local anesthetic.

It is always advisable to have a first aid kit to anticipate first aid treatment. Because it is so difficult to find nontoxic supplies, it is a "must" for the allergic person.

Warning: Although Dr. Eloise Kailin helped prepare this list for her most sensitive patients, it is important for you who have the problem

179

to be very careful to check this entire approach with your own doctor. *No product is safe for everyone. No procedure is safe for everyone.*

FIRST AID KIT

Acetylsalicylic Acid, Pure. Five grains in clear gelatin capsule (*if* aspirin is tolerated). This is corn-free aspirin. When an aspirin is needed, empty the contents of capsule in teaspoon.

Alkali Salts. As with any medical procedure, first consult with your doctor.

Order two parts sodium bicarbonate to one part potassium bicarbonate, chemically pure. Some druggists order by the pound and will let you mix the ingredients. Others will prepare small bottles with the correct mixture. WARNING: ALKALI SALTS CANNOT BE USED BY HEART PATIENTS WHO MUST LIMIT SALT (SODIUM) INTAKE. Such people must rely on Milk of Magnesia: one to two teaspoons for alkalinization.

Use as a laxative and to offset food and some chemical exposures. Do not use more than twice a week without consulting your doctor. Use with caution if swollen ankles or puffy eyes indicate water retention.

Antihistamine. Of course, it is not up to us to recommend any medication. Use what is prescribed by your physician. Substitute any other anti-allergic medicine, also prescribed by your physician. However, we can recommend a special preparation of antihistamine (see Medications).

Baking Soda. Arm & Hammer brand seems to be tolerated well.

Hot Water Bottle. Use pure gum latex for nonrubber sensitive patient.

Hydrogen Peroxide. 3 percent strength for surface wounds.

Infra Red Light Bulb, Holder. For local heat, if sensitive to hot water bottle.

Irrigation Can. Enamel with hard rubber attachments. Tubing to be pure gum latex or rubber, whichever is best tolerated by the individual. For douche or enemas.

Medications. When special drugs must be prescribed, it is often possible to obtain them free of dyes, starches, gums, and other potential allergens by asking the doctor to specify the injectable form of the drug to be added to distilled water (stored in a glass container) so that it can be taken orally. Keep in refrigerator as it is preservative-free.

Become acquainted with a pharmacist who will understand the need for extra care in his technique in the preparation of drugs, and who will prepare medications in glass containers instead of plastic.

Milk of Magnesia. Plain, liquid; do not use flavored or tablet form.

Surgex Tube Gauze. It comes in six sizes, fingers, toes, head, shoulders, arms, and legs. Because you can twist it, you don't need an adhesive tape. It should not be placed in direct contact with the body because it is treated. As a layer over pure gauze, however, it can be used by some very sensitive people. Plain cotton bandage can be substituted.

Thermometer. Any glass thermometer is satisfactory.

Triangular Bandage. Cotton or unbleached muslin, prewashed to remove sizing so that it will be ready for use.

Two Trays of Ice. After freezing, remove ice from tray and place in a glass jar in a conspicuous place in the freezer. (For those sensitive to chlorine, use spring water to make ice.) The ice is important for local application, as described below.

Zephiran. Zephiran chloride, aqueous solution 1:750 (for antiseptic use). Avoid tinctured zephiran which contains a dye.

FIRST AID TREATMENT

Allergic Reaction. If the causative allergen is a food eaten not over an hour prior to reaction, try to induce vomiting by putting finger in the throat to induce gagging. If vomiting is not possible, take a laxative dose of milk of magnesia, four tablespoons (for adult) taken with one pint of water. Drink another pint of water within an hour.

For other reactions, such as fume exposure, use prescribed antihistamines and other anti-allergic medication prescribed. Or take one half teaspoon of alkali salts in a glass of water. Follow with a minimum of one quart of water. If nausea and vomiting do not permit oral medication, take one pint of spring water enema to which has been added one teaspoon of alkali salts. Retain it as long as possible. When salts are not allowed, a pint of plain spring water may be used.

Take oxygen as prescribed.

Bee Stings. Apply ice cube at site of sting. Take alkali salts. If there is a serious reaction on an arm or leg (swelling or itching on parts of the body distant from the sting), apply tourniquet to prevent rapid absorption. For a sting on head, neck, or body, apply ice cube. Severe reactions with shock or breathing disturbance may require an emergency ambulance. Other preventive measures may be prescribed by physician if previous reaction was treated. Some very sensitive people have found great relief from large doses of vitamin C. Consult with the physician for suggested dosage.

Burns. It is important to recognize the degree of burns.

first degree:	redness only
second degree:	blisters
third degree:	deep burns, severe pain, nerve ends destroyed.

Since the chemically sensitive person has a particular problem with infections, be extremely cautious with both second- and third-degree burns. *Consult your doctor.*

Speed is an important factor in treating burns to reduce heat in the tissues as fast as possible. Put burned part into cold water *immediately* using ice cubes only if immediately at hand. Pour cold water (spring water for those who are sensitive) over ice cubes to loosen. Pour the ice water into a bowl and use for soaking the burn. Use the loosened cubes to keep the water cold until the burning sensation subsides.

If burning feeling persists, apply soupy paste made of bicarbonate of soda and spring water, or use cold compresses. When dry, use firm bandages of clean cotton flannel held in place by gauze. If not sensitive to tea, use concentrated solution of tea applied directly to burn.

Chemical Exposures. It is advisable to wash your hair and shower as soon as you return home from a bout with heavy traffic, a smoke-filled room, or an exposure to perfume. Just by shaking hands with someone who is wearing perfume, you may find the odor clinging to your person and your clothes. If you can't launder it immediately, put your clothing in the basement.

Colds. Is it a cold or an allergic reaction? The mucus from nose or throat seldom remains clear over thirty-six hours in the presence of bacterial infection, but with an allergic reaction, mucus is usually clear.

Try to observe whether the color of your nasal mucus is clear like water, white like paper, or yellow. If it is often yellow without other signs of illness, you will not be able to determine if you have a cold. However, if your allergic reactions are usually accompanied only by clear mucus, you can be reasonably certain that colored or dark mucus indicates a cold.

The same holds true for an elevated temperature. If reactions are accompanied by a high temperature, you may need a doctor to diagnose a cold. If, however, your temperature remains normal during most reactions, you can assume an elevated temperature, along with other cold symptoms, means the fever of a cold.

What to do: Drink one cup of hot water, gulped every waking hour while throat is sore. Use other medication such as antihistamine or vitamin C in large doses, as prescribed by your doctor. Take ½ teaspoon of alkali salts with a full glass of water. Get plenty of rest. Drink as much water as you can.

Aspirin (pure acetylsalicylic acid), if tolerated, may be used for ache, temperature, or discomfort. Remember, it cures nothing. Besides, a moderately elevated temperature helps trigger your defenses against infection. When you need to telephone your doctor, be prepared to tell him your pulse and temperature.

A very bad allergic reaction that resembles a cold weakens your resistance and makes you more susceptible to a bacterial infection.

Constipation. Spring water enemas may be used. For long-term use, do not take more than one enema a week without checking with your doctor.

Cuts. Cleanse with hydrogen peroxide or aqueous Zephiran solution, 1:750. Cover with firm cotton bandage secured with cotton gauze.

Effective Vaporizer. Use a Corningware coffee pot, with a tent over it made from a towel, and breathe in the vapors. Be sure to use plain spring water (your drinking water). Remove the top of the pot if it is Bakelite.

Insect Stings and Bites. Vinegar eases the pain of most stings or bites and is particularly soothing on sunburn as well. Here again, consult with the doctor about vitamin C, which has helped many people.

Rashes and Itching. Pat milk of magnesia on affected area. If rash is in a moist, sweaty area, it may be dusted with any allowed starch powder such as arrowroot, potato, or rice starch.

Sore Throat. Gulping hot water is most effective. For relief, gargle with one teaspoon of vinegar, if tolerated, in a cup of water. Consult with your physician about massive doses of vitamin C.

Steam. When steam is required, spring water in a Pyrex tea or coffee pot may be safely inhaled if care is taken to prevent scalding. Some people can tolerate the hard Bakelite units which sit in glass containers for overnight steam production. These should be the kind that shut off when the water runs out.

Sprains. To relieve sprain discomfort, use cold applications for the first twenty-four hours. After that, use hot applications.

CHAPTER 22

Educating the Medical Practitioner

Whenative consider that less than a hundred years ago a patient burning with fever was denied a drop of water because it was considered lethal for his condition, it is not surprising that a pioneer field such as clinical ecology is having its own struggles to win acceptance.

However, many of the doctors who at one time scoffed at this medical innovation, or questioned its value, have become its most enthusiastic practitioners. Some were motivated to try it because of a personal insoluble health problem suffered either by themselves or by some member of their immediate family.

In spite of the fact that they were doctors, they had the same difficulties that many of you may now be experiencing, both in finding a correct diagnosis of their complaints and suitable treatment for them, and in suffering from chronic illness and finding no answer through conventional medical channels.

A number of these doctors have been willing to share their personal experiences. We feel sure that many of you will identify with the stories that follow.

Dr. X's problem first became apparent to him when he was chief of thoracic surgery at a Veterans Administration Hospital. He found he was having difficulty staying awake while driving; he kept falling asleep at the wheel.

He had frequent bouts of the flu, frequent spells of dizziness, and once, nearly blacked out as he was leaving surgery. A colleague helped him to a chair. Dr. X told his colleague that this was not the first time and proceeded to describe the problems he'd been having. The colleague, an eye, ear, nose, and throat specialist suggested Dr. X see an allergist. The shots recommended by the allergist gave some relief, but only for a short time. Dr. X realized he had to look further.

A chance meeting with a former medical student of his resulted in Dr. X's taking the series of innovative food tests discussed in Chapter 2. Unfortunately, even though he now knew the complexity of his

184

problem, Dr. X knew of no allergist who accepted the validity of the food tests, so no treatment could result.

He began to do extensive reading on the subject. He learned that he is a universal food reactor; that is, all foods give him some difficulty in varying degrees. He deals with this by abstaining from food all during his long working day, eating only when he gets home, and adhering strictly to his rotary diet.

Dr. X also learned about chemical sensitivity resulting from the environment. This led to the realization that chemical sensitivity might be his problem as well. His next step was to attempt to remove all chemical excitants from his environment. This involved drastic changes in his home—removing gas heaters, gas stove, and gas boiler, plus other pollutants like rugs—all of which was mind-boggling to his wife.

Even so, his health did not show substantial improvement until he was able to alter his work environment as well. The more toxins he removed, the more his health improved. At this point, Dr. X's health is not only better than it has been since his problem began, but actually better than he can ever remember it. He no longer has colds and no longer falls asleep over the evening newspaper. Now this doctor, who had barely enough energy to take him through his work day, has energy for all kinds of family pursuits whenever he has free time.

Dr. X's case has many ramifications. His awareness of his own problem has made him more observant of the reaction of some of his heart patients. This has led him to recognize the full impact of the environment on cardiovascular disorders. His practice has expanded to include clinical ecology and he now teaches his heart patients how to cope with the pollution in their environment.

Another doctor, Dr. L, who suffered some of the same symptoms as Dr. X, namely, flu, fatigue, aches, and pains, also had other symptoms which led him to consult one specialist after another, an internist, a urologist, an orthopedic surgeon. In each case, the specialist could find no illness in his particular field of expertise. Dr. L told us that he would be dead today if he had not stumbled onto a clinical ecologist.

To quote Dr. L, "I was not able to think, or to work, I suffered from constant pains. When I mentioned my numerous symptoms to the clinical ecologist, he told me that I was probably suffering from ecologic disease. I thought that was the most stupid statement I had heard in twenty years.

"And yet no doctor had been able to help me and I continued to suffer from urinary difficulties, back pain, chest pain, fatigue, depression, mental confusion, and disgraphia [transposing numbers].

"As it turned out, ecologic disease was not so stupid-sounding as I thought—clinical ecology has revolutionized my life. When I am in my oasis, my good environment, I feel well."

The testing changed Dr. L's life. As he told us, "As a result of testing, I had to change my whole life style. I had to give up hospital practice entirely. Clinical ecology has changed my practice of medicine by alerting me to the fact that I am sensitive to hospitals.

"I think American hospitals today are one of the most contaminated single sources of environmental pollution. They have the plastic odors, sprays, perfumes, deodorants, smoking, bath soaps, carpeting, chemical solutions from operating rooms, all being recirculated through centralized air conditioning. American hospitals are bad."

The practice of clinical ecology does not take place exclusively in the United States. There is the case of an English physician, Dr. O, who had written a book on low carbohydrate diets. Inadvertently, he discovered that people on this diet were showing signs of relief from other health problems, which indicated to him that avoiding carbohydrates can cure more than just obesity.

As a result, he accepted the advice of a colleague and paid a visit to Dr. Theron Randolph in Chicago. Randolph pointed out the missing link: by avoiding carbohydrates, people are also avoiding grains. Since so many people are allergic to grains, the low carbohydrate diet alleviated some of their allergic symptoms. While in Chicago, Dr. O also learned that not only grains but other foods and many chemicals cause problems.

Dr. O's experience reinforces our belief that there is a common factor in many of the crash diets and fad diets that seem to help people temporarily. It is possible that people are losing weight not because of the diet per se but because they are avoiding foods they are allergic to.

Dr. O applied in his medical practice what he had learned from Dr. Randolph. He discovered that for him the main application was psychiatric, since he was interested in cerebral allergy. He became a psychiatrist in order to help people who had been misdiagnosed, who were suffering psychiatric disorders caused by the environment and/or foods.

It's interesting to note a personal bonus for Dr. O. Since he became involved in this program, he has been able to detect that gasoline fumes and oil products cause depression in him.

Dr. E, another psychiatrist, found help for his whole family as a result of a chance meeting with two famous clinical ecologists.

"For a number of years," he says, "I had some peculiar symptoms involving the left side of my body. I consulted neurologists, neurosurgeons, and had exhaustive neurological workups at a university hospital.

"They could not come up with a diagnosis. I also had symptoms that I called 'anxiety attacks' that I later came to understand were withdrawal reactions from a corn addiction. This led me to get interested in the subject of relative hypoglycemia.

"Being a psychiatrist, I happened to attend a psychiatric meeting at which Dr. Randolph and Dr. Rea were speakers. I found their ideas intriguing.

"Because of my symptoms and the increasing awareness that I had a problem, particularly with foods, I decided to be self-admitted to Dr. Rea's ecologic unit in Dallas. I had what I think was a rare opportunity to be both patient and colleague to Dr. Rea and made rounds with him, seeing patients, and learning a great deal about my own sensitivities and those of others. All the symptoms that had plagued me for twenty-one years were revealed, by testing, to be allergic in nature, involving the vessels on the left side of my body.

"I subsequently sent my sister, who for twenty years we believed had had multiple sclerosis. I had my daughter down there and found there was familial incidence of vasculitis [an inherited blood vessel abnormality].

"After I discovered that these factors produced symptoms that I had been treating with psychotherapy, unsuccessfully, for a number of years, I had to change the nature of my practice and took clinical ecology into my psychiatric practice. I now am enjoying the practice of medicine much more and feel that I am benefiting more people in that practice.

"My sister has improved symptomatically. She had problems with fatigue, memory, obesity, balance, urinary symptoms of frequency and poor control, thought to be part of the multiple sclerosis. After she was worked up ecologically, her problem with control and leakage of urine improved significantly. She also has had no further acute attacks requiring hospitalization."

Granted, food allergies and sensitivities are difficult to diagnose unless they are unmasked. Because clinical ecology is not yet taught in medical schools, doctors aren't trained to look for the symptoms. That training is very important. The late Dr. Herbert Rinkel had this axiom for doctors: "One must be taught to suspect, for if one does not suspect, he does not test and if he does not test, he does not know."

The importance of this axiom is demonstrated in the case of Dr. G., who had a marked tendency to fall asleep throughout his years in medical school. It was particularly troublesome in the late morning. Before his most important lecture at 10:30 A.M., he would drink three cups of coffee to help him stay awake. Because he hated coffee, he ate doughnuts or French pastry with it. Nothing helped.

He told us this story because no one paid any attention to his symptoms. As he puts it, "I am sure that the long array of professors were quite aware of that guy asleep somewhere in that lecture hall.

"No one came up to me to suggest, 'Hey, have you ever thought you might have hypoglycemia?' Nobody ever said, 'Have you checked to see if you have any cerebral allergies? Narcolepsy?' Even if they weren't astute enough to know about food allergies, at least they could say, 'Maybe you're narcoleptic.'

"Years later," he recounted, "I had my testing with Marshall Mandell. When he put wheat drops under my tongue, in a few minutes my ears turned red and my tongue got so thick I couldn't speak well.

"We laughed about it, but again in a few minutes, I fell asleep. Now it was proven conclusively—it was the wheat that made me fall asleep."

We have included these cases involving physicians who are patients, to show you that even doctors with the problem have had difficulties finding someone knowledgeable in this field. After *you* have been tested by a clinical ecologist, there will be times when you will need to consult with doctors for problems unrelated to your allergies and sensitivities—dentists, opthalmologists, surgeons, and others. Be prepared to explain your problem, but proceed with caution lest the uninitiated medical man jumps to the conclusion that you are neurotic and need a psychiatrist.

Avoid a lengthy detailed explanation to the doctor who is a stranger to the problem of multiple chemical intolerances. Instead, introduce the subject by presenting your clinical allergist's check list prepared in conjunction with Medic Alert. It is then safe to answer any of the doctor's questions. The open-minded, forward-thinking physician will be willing to cooperate with you and consult your referring clinical ecologist.

If, however, the doctor is derisive and pooh-poohs the idea, you would probably be wise to ask your clinical ecologist to recommend another physician known to be more understanding of the problem. Don't wait for an emergency before finding an understanding physician. Establish the necessary rapport with a doctor during a routine checkup. Above all, don't let shyness or awe of the doctor deter you because the consequences can be very grave.

"More and more the patient is coming to realize that he or she has the final say about what is going to be done with his or her body," says Dr. Michael Schachter of Nyack, New York, a psychiatrist who has turned to orthomolecular psychiatry and clinical ecology. "Therefore, if things are recommended that he knows are going to be harmful to him, then he should turn down the recommendation and find another physician.

"It is a delicate problem, to tell one doctor about what another is doing, but the patient has the right to find out whether the doctor knows of particular work that is going on in the medical field which is of special importance to that patient.

"Perhaps the patient could say something like this, 'Look, this is something written by another physician doing this work and I have found it has been very helpful to me. I would appreciate it if you would familiarize yourself with it a little bit so we can talk the same language. I understand (or, in my reading I realize) that some of this is not getting into the orthodox medical literature, but it seems to work for me.'

"Thus, without getting on a high-horse and insulting him, the patient can open the doctor's mind a bit. The patient has to strike a balance between coming on too strongly in a know-it-all fashion on one hand, and not being too intimidated on the other hand.

"As the patient learns more about allergies and his or her own condition, it will be easier to strike the balance between firmness and a willingness to learn more."

The most encouraging message that we have for you is that more and more doctors are starting to test patients for allergies before operating to remove various organs of the body, knowing, for example, that gall bladder symptoms can be brought on by food allergies.

It is our hope that more doctors will explore the ecological approach to medicine so that they can include it in their own practice or at least become knowledgeable enough to refer their patients to a clinical ecologist.

PART V

A Practical Guide to Nontoxic Living

CHAPTER 23

Housing: Where to Live and How to Live There

ALICE, a woman who had reached the acute stage of allergic reaction moved six times before deciding that she must build her own home according to the specifications of her doctor. In order to make her environment free from indoor pollution, she followed all the suggestions made by her doctor (that is, all she could afford).

When she finally moved into her home, her state of health improved to such an extent that she felt she might be able to return to work eventually, even though her doctors had originally told her she would never again be able to be gainfully employed.

As her health improved, Alice was very happy that she had selected a place far enough out in the country to avoid heavy pollution, but close enough to the city so that she would be able to commute, if her health improved enough that she could return to work.

Unfortunately, there was one very important aspect that she had overlooked—progress. Just as her health was improving, construction began on a four-lane highway, which would pass within five hundred yards of her home. So close was the highway she could smell the fumes of the machines that were plowing up the dirt. When told of her problem the construction crew was most considerate and gave her as much advance notice as possible before tarring the road, so that she could make arrangements to leave her home and seek refuge elsewhere.

Sad but true, there were very few ecologically safe places to which she could escape. Many times during the building of the road she became very ill, and called the construction foreman to discover that the crew was working on something they thought would not affect her and so had not notified her.

Once when Alice became ill, she called the foreman who was astonished at the degree of her sensitivity. He told her that a small area of the road had to be corrected, and he had not notified her because they were tarring this surface more than two miles from her home. The site of this house had been chosen because the prevailing winds blew across fields filled with trees, far from any roads. There were such good cross winds that when she opened her windows on days that were not polluted, she was able to have good fresh air in her home. The sad part of this story is that once the road was completed and traffic became heavy, the fumes were so intolerable that rarely during the day could she open her windows. Her greatest fear now is that the traffic will become so heavy that she will have to move from the home that had given her so much hope for future good health.

We repeat her story so you will not make the same mistakes she did. Before selecting the site for a new home, make sure that you check with the authorities to find out if there are any plans for new roads, or for plants and factories whose chemicals could pollute your environment.

Having carefully selected your home site, be sure that your builder follows your instructions to the letter. If not, you might experience a problem similar to that of Thomas, a gentleman who thought his new house was ecologically sound and free from indoor pollution.

When his cousin Charlotte came to visit Thomas in his new home, she complained about an unpleasant odor that was particularly noticeable in his bedroom, and which made her nauseous. Since the floors were pure wood, and there was nothing in the bedroom except a carefully selected bed, Thomas examined the closet to see if the odor was coming from the shelves. He found that pressed board shelving had been substituted for the pure wood he had requested. The glue used in the process of manufacturing the pressed board was so toxic that it permeated the house.

The strange thing about all of this is that Charlotte, who had always made light of allergies, detected the offending odor while Thomas did not. There is a simple explanation. As a result of his illness Thomas had lost his sense of smell. Charlotte was able to detect it because she came from a contaminated environment into his pure environment which heightened her sense of smell.

This experience reminded Charlotte that she always felt nauseated in her own home and had been unable to figure out why. They decided to check her closet shelves and found the same toxic shelving material. The skeptic became a believer.

Test. If you suspect something in your house is bothering you, go for a brisk two-hour walk. When you reenter your home, the first thing you react to—remove it!

Obviously, not everyone can build or even buy a home, but if you rent a home or an apartment, there are things you can do to improve your environment. One word of caution: *If you are renting, have an escape clause in your lease.* If the environment makes you ill, you can then move upon furnishing a note from your doctor.

Just because you are renting, however, don't skip over the following section as unimportant to you. There are many changes you can make that are not costly, such as changing an air-conditioning filter. Also, many changes are available that involve improvements you can take with you wherever you move. For example, you could buy portable baseboard heaters. These allow you to turn off hot-air heat and convert to baseboard heat without investing in your landlord's property.

PLANNING A HOUSE

Air Conditioning. Central air-conditioning units should be surrounded by materials that can be tolerated. Units without insulation can be obtained directly from the factory. Since air conditioners are manufactured only during the winter, the order must be placed well in advance.

Bathrooms. Plastic and synthetic compositions are now used for all kinds of bathroom fixtures. Request a wooden toilet seat, a porcelain sink, and a porcelain tub. Make sure the base of the shower stall is tile and not a plasticized substitute for cement. The bathroom floor, as well as the stall-shower floor, should be made of the 4″ × 4″ tile rather than small tile. The same flooring should be used in the powder room. Avoid plastic shower units. All plumbing should be copper or galvanized piping.

Bathroom Towel Racks. It is necessary to have enough towel racks to spread out wet towels so they will dry more quickly. If towels have to be folded on the rack there is a greater chance of mold developing. Don't leave the number up to the builder; he will never provide enough racks.

Near every stall shower an extra towel rack should be placed to hold large pieces of toweling that can be used to dry down the sides and floor of the shower. There should also be a towel rack so that a bath mat can be hung up to dry. This is most important, especially if you are sensitive to mold.

Bedroom. We'd like to emphasize that it is a good idea to sleep in a very small room containing only your bed, and use an adjoining or other separate room as a dressing room where you keep your clothes. Your bed should be in a room by itself so you do not have to inhale fumes from the rest of the area; there should be as many windows as possible and those windows should not face onto a street or any other place where there are cars or other fumes.

Cabinets and Counter Tops. Be sure that you have the original Formica. As you become more and more involved with pure living, you will find that you are doing more and more cooking. Therefore, it is advisable to look ahead and plan your counter tops accordingly.

You will find that Corningware chopping boards are valuable tools. For those who already have a house built, it will be necessary to buy these separately. The largest size, 16″ × 20″, is recommended. When you are building a new home, it is recommended that you have two or three of these chopping boards placed permanently in strategic places in your counter tops.

As for the cabinets, they can be made of Formica, wood, metal, or even stone or ceramic tile. A major concern is to watch out for synthetic glues or stains. Many houses are contaminated by the use of commercial stains. Use walnut shells to make a nontoxic stain. Grind up the walnut shells, add water, and boil until the water changes color. It makes an excellent stain but is difficult to keep clean. (If you have scratches on your furniture you can rub them out by using a piece of walnut or pecan. The raw wood will absorb the stain from the nut.)

Carpeting. Carpeting is not recommended because it is too great a contaminant to the environment. Besides being a dust and mold collector, it adds fumes that make your environment impure.

Caulking. Use DAP. *Avoid all silicone caulking;* this kind of caulking never loses its toxicity. Be very careful to get the old tub & tile DAP. The new foam DAP is very toxic.

Cement. Calcium chloride should not be added to any ready-mix cement. No quick-drying agent should be added.

Closet Doors. A sliding door is not recommended, but if you must use sliding doors, ask for wood or metal handles, not plastic. You need a door that can be closed completely, if there are items in your closet that might cause a problem. Every closet should have a fan so it can be aired from time to time.

Copper Pipes. Copper piping is controversial, for it is now believed that people are absorbing enough copper from their drinking water to cause a zinc deficiency. Copper pipes, however, still are one of the two best kinds of pipes available.

We recommend that when drawing water for drinking or cooking, make sure that the water runs for five minutes, if it hasn't been turned on for several hours.

Galvanized pipes, when obtainable, are the best choice. Of course, you must never use plastic pipes for water that will be used for drinking or cooking.

Dishwashers. From the standpoint of avoiding toxicity the best dishwasher is one that has a stainless steel interior. Waste King makes one.

Doors. Unless you are going to use carpeting—and we strongly advise against it—make sure that when doors are measured, they are not shortened to allow for carpeting. Because carpeting is so often included in a new house, builders automatically cut off approximately an inch from the bottom of the door to allow for carpeting. If you find that inch of space between the floor and the bottom of the door, it will make that room harder to seal off from the rest of the house.

Say you want to have a storeroom for objects that affect you, or that you want to close off one of the children's rooms because it is cluttered with dust-collecting toys and books. If you have space underneath the door, fumes will come in. Make sure the builders do not shorten your doors.

Frequently, houses are planned with archways instead of doorways. Whenever possible, substitute with doors. This is especially important in the kitchen to prevent odors from spreading to the rest of the house.

Make sure that storage space in the basement is separated from the rest of the area by a solid door.

Dryer, Washing Machine. When you are buying a dryer and a washing machine for your home, make sure that you have an outdoor vent for the dryer. The salespeople may tell you that it is not absolutely necessary; however, one woman noticed dampness around her dryer and thought the machine was faulty. When she called the shop from which she had purchased the dryer, she was told it was because she did not have an outside vent. This dampness causes mold.

Electric Fixtures. We recommend that in the process of building, you have recessed fixtures put in the ceiling, even in rooms where you don't usually find them, for example, in the living room. It is one of the best ways to have lighting that is easily cleaned, does not collect dust, and reduces the number of lamps needed.

Electricity. When wiring the house for electricity, anticipate having an extra load. After moving in, some persons with allergies have put in an extra freezer or even an extra oven. During the initial period, those who cannot tolerate heated metal may wish to cook in the basement. Later, they may choose to continue to cook there to avoid odors in the kitchen.

Electric Outlets. Just as you have to allow for enough electricity, so it is important that you have enough electric outlets. Place outlets in strategic spots where you may not ordinarily find them. Have extra plugs for extra refrigerators, freezers, or even stoves in your basement. Have extra outlets on the patio or even in a screened-in area for outdoor cooking. Some homes have just one or two outlets in the bathroom. At the time you are building, it does not cost much to have more put in, but it is a large expense if you install them after your home is completed.

Plugs are vulnerable to contamination because air comes through them. Plaster around the outlets. Also, try to get metal plugs rather than plastic ones. They cost a little more but are worth it, because they do not contaminate the air.

Exterior Walls and Trim. Have exterior walls constructed of brick. The exterior trim should be natural wood, not plastic. Stormguard, zinc-coated nails will not stain the wood.

Fans. If you have a large attic fan, a permanently sealed motor is desirable. It is useful for quickly removing smoke and other contaminants from the house. Fans can be used in closets and cabinets to carry off fumes from various motors and offensive materials stored inside the house. A basement fan with an outdoor exhaust is helpful in preventing mold and musty odors. It would be a marvelous idea to have one fan on every floor, but the top floor and basement are the most important.

Fans have made it possible for some sensitive people to have a self-cleaning oven, although Dr. Eloise Kailin recommends against it. When using the oven open the window in the kitchen, turn on the kitchen and upstairs fans and keep them on all the time the self-cleaning oven is on.

It is true that it is still necessary for some sensitive people to leave the house for forty-eight hours. However, without fans, sensitive people can detect oven fumes as long as a week later. Continuous cleaning ovens should not be used under any conditions.

Floors. These types of floors are recommended: brick, hardwood, stone, terrazzo, cement, terra cotta. Some people can tolerate vinyl floors. "CMC" 348 Emulsion adhesive has been used successfully by some patients in installing vinyl tile. This is a resin emulsion that comes in five-gallon cans. Asbestos tile, plastic linoleums or tiles, and finishes on hardwood floors are not recommended.

Armstrong inlaid linoleum flooring has been found to be satisfactory in the kitchen, but cannot be used in the basement. If you have a finished cement floor, warn your builder in advance that you need a smooth finish which can be used as a play area for shuffleboard, and other games, thus turning a minus into a plus.

If you find a kitchen flooring you can tolerate, we recommend using the same material for steps, dining room, and halls. Hardwood floors are difficult to clean, if they are untreated and have no varnish.

Fluorescent Lighting. It is a no-no, it gives off ozone.

Formica. Formica can be used because it is a very hard plastic. Usually old Bakelite is all right also, except for the most sensitive patients.

Do not let the builder use a synthetic Formica substitute for the countertop and dressing table in your bathroom. For those who are extremely sensitive, it is advisable that two layers of Formica be used so that the glue is between the layers and is less likely to affect you.

Foundation. Cement block in place of cinder block for the foundation works well. Many other light-weight building blocks resembling cinder blocks have a synthetic base.

Frame. Fir lumber can be used for framing material.

Garage. Must be separate from house, not under the same roof.

Heating. Heating is the biggest problem in building a new ecologic house or converting an old one. In the past, any electric heat was used and thought to be safe, but now clinical ecologists are finding out that some people are sensitive to electric heat, specifically hot-air heat. Gas and oil heating units are the least desirable. Forced air heat of any kind should be avoided.

Solar heating should be investigated as the first source. It has been suggested that even if you are in an area where you have to have a secondary system, the expenses of heating your house will be minimized. It is worth your while to investigate it.

Dr. William Rea recommends that for new homes hot-water heat in copper coils or copper pipes be installed under terrazzo floors. Terrazzo is a good nontoxic flooring substance.

Do not put heat ducts in a floor with vinyl or other synthetics around them. It is also wise to put heat ducts in ceilings to heat the floor above.

Low temperature types of electric baseboard heat are recommended because they do not give off gas or oil fumes, there is no chance of a cracked firebox, and the low heat does not scorch lint and dust on the unit.

It is important that the materials used do not give off noxious fumes. Copper radiators are best, and the baseboard should be made of steel. Copper radiators with aluminum baseboards or vents are also available.

It is common knowledge that many people are sensitive to silver and gold jewelry. What is not well known is that many are also sensitive to aluminum, nickel, iron, and stainless steel. For some people, the primary sensitivity is actual contact with the metal. For others, the reaction is to the fumes, especially when these metals are heated.

Some can tolerate aluminum when it is not being used for cooking, but the minute it is heated, have a problem with it. Others can tolerate the odor of the burners on an electric stove only when they are not heated. The minute the heat is on, even at low temperature, they get a reaction.

Some persons have resorted to extreme means to get away from irritants in the house. One man started sleeping outside in a sleeping bag, using an umbrella to keep snow off his face. He considered it a great housing improvement to sleep in a metal storage room in the back yard. When he finally got a plumber to remove the gas furnace, he replaced it with electric heat. Making a clean sweep of the toxic materials in his house, he replaced rugs with hardwood floors to which he was not allergic. Even so, it took about a year for all evidence of the excitants to be gone from the house, before he could move back in.

For those who are interested in baseboard heating but are sensitive to metal there is a solution. A plumber, who has the problem himself, and has helped many people, told us that many people can better tolerate this system of heating if they put in twice as many units as are required under normal circumstances. In that way the heating is spread over a greater number of units, and the fixtures themselves do not become heated to such a high degree.

One of the problems of baseboard heating units is that they are dust collectors. However, they are supposed to be detachable, so that you can remove the outer protective metal and get into the mechanism with a vacuum cleaner to remove the dust. In planning your home, make sure that the plumber as well as the builder and the workmen who put in molding and floors are aware that you want these units to be detachable.

A gas heater with the boiler outside the house is acceptable with baseboard heat; so is a coal heater with the boiler outside. Electric heat, with radiators or coils inside the house, is more often acceptable.

It is a good idea to have the boiler about twelve feet from the house, so that the only thing pumped into the house is hot water, enclosed in pipes. It is important that the pipes be underground and insulated so that they will not burst in subzero weather.

Duct work insulation for heat and air conditioning should be placed on the outside of ducts; only aluminum foil insulation is acceptable.

Heaters. International Hot Water electric baseboard heating units can be stripped of all rubber and plastic parts. The manufacturer will perform this service. Be sure to contact, in advance, the main office for this service.[1] These can be installed or remain portable.

Some of the electric baseboard heating units are coated with a plastic which soon burns off. These units are preferable to those that are tar-coated.

Humidity. Before putting in any kind of electrical equipment for removing humidity, or for anything involved in moisture, aside from concern over mold, you must be concerned with the instruments that give off ozone. We don't know of any safe method.

Insulation. When choosing insulation you will need an aluminum barrier. Use yellow fiberglass instead of red fiberglass. It must have an aluminum paper shield. In no case use urethane foam. Place insulation on outside of ducts, not inside. Reinforced aluminum instead of plastic sheets can be placed over insulation behind plastic board. Fiberglass without the vapor barrier may be the best solution if it is covered with heavy-duty aluminum foil.

Interior Trim. Wood or Formica should be used for all cabinet work. Glass wall shelves can be used in the kitchen. All molding should be wood.

Lamps. You are probably accustomed to your own lamps but if you have to replace them, you may find out how much the wiring bothered you. Once lamps are two to four years old they are not so troublesome, but if you have to replace them, it may be difficult to find lamps that you can tolerate. If you have ceiling fixtures, then there is no wiring problem.

Lighting. Any glass, metal, or pewter fixtures may be used. Recessed incandescent bulbs may be used with a metal grill. This minimizes the need for styrofoams, fiberglass, and other synthetics.

Outdoor Plugs. It is important to have enough outside electrical sockets, because when you live in a clear environment you may find the advantage of not using the stove in your kitchen. If you are one of those people affected by heated metal, you may be affected by your oven and by electrical equipment inside the house. Some of your appliances may bother you even if you are not aware of it, so you may want to use your juicer and other small appliances outside, on a patio.

Outdoor Storage. This can be incorporated in a courtyard designed to house articles not tolerated, such as guests' coats or printed matter.

Ovens. For those people who are sensitive to metal it is recommended that you buy a Corningware range oven. This is a range that has a top of Corning glassware. One patient reported that it was easy to clean and a marvelous way to cook. Other ranges imitating the Corningware are now on the market. They may be satisfactory, but we have not received any word on these.

Paint. Some highly sensitive patients have found they can enter a house four to eight days after it has been painted, if Dupont Lucite without Teflon has been used. Some people have found they respond even better if they mix one box of baking soda to a gallon of the Dupont Lucite without Teflon. This method has been used satisfactorily in a comprehensive environmentally controlled unit in a hospital for people with this problem. Keep adding baking soda to the paint until the bubbling action stops.

Avoid premixed paint because it has Teflon in it. The manufacturer does not put Teflon in the tint base.

We don't believe in using tints, for the dyes will have fixatives that are toxic. Walls should be either off-white or white, but not stark white. A little pigment is needed to keep tint base from being so white it almost hurts your eyes.

Paneling. Paneling should be of pure wood. If it isn't hardwood, be very careful of it because it is usually loaded with formaldehyde. If it is pure wood, do not glue it in; use nails.

Pantry. Besides having a large window in the kitchen—which helps to get rid of some of the fumes from the freezer and refrigerator—it is recommended you have a special pantry with a window and door closing it off from the kitchen so you won't get the odors from those two large appliances. Have a fan installed in the pantry to draw out the fumes.

Plaster and Grout. It is important to use plaster that has not been treated. It should contain no quick-drying agents or any other agents. Test it before using to be sure that it does not affect you. Grouting should be plain with no coloring agents in it. Make sure there is no sealer.

Refrigerator. Select an electric refrigerator with a minimum of plastic-coated wiring. Do not use a self-defrosting type of refrigerator.

For the most sensitive, porcelain or steel refrigerators are best. These are commercial refrigerators and cannot be found in the home appliance areas of department stores. A word of caution, however: Do not get a high-humidity commercial refrigerator. This machine is dripping wet inside, because it is designed to keep dough damp.

If possible, you should not have the motor of the refrigerator in the house. The motor can be installed outside and the current piped in using glycol rather than Freon. The reason for using glycol is that if you have a leak you will know it immediately, because glycol is a liquid. Freon is a gaseous refrigerant which, when leaking, often goes undetected.

If you cannot have a stainless steel or porcelain refrigerator, keep your refrigerator extra cold. It is wise never to keep food without a cover in a refrigerator.

If you must have a refrigerator with a motor in it, you should not have it in the kitchen, but in another room, closed off, with a vent to the outside. Once you begin to be aware of the fact you are reacting to them, you can more easily pinpoint contaminants. You may decide you want an extra refrigerator or an extra freezer in your basement.

Roof. Slate shingle, wood shingle, ceramic tile, metal shingle, or metal roofing are all satisfactory materials. For flat roofs, the combination of tar and gravel may be acceptable in place of tar, and probably will not create difficulty after volatizing (aging).

Screens. Would you believe it? Manufacturers are now making screens from fiberglass. Insist on metal screens.

Showers. When selecting a door for a shower, make sure that you choose one with hinges rather than the sliding door which has grooves. Water accumulates in the grooves and causes a mold problem. This is why a stall shower is more advisable than a shower added to a tub.

Stove. A Corningware stove is truly a delight, eliminating the bothersome fumes from formaldehyde coating on regular burners.

Stove Hoods. A stove should be double-vented above. An extra-powerful vent is important and, if possible, the stove, refrigerator, and dishwasher should be shut off completely from the rest of the room with solid doors that enclose the area. Thermodor makes an oven which has its own vent.

Swimming Pools. Don't have one unless you can have one that does not use chlorine.

Telephones. When you have your telephone installed, make sure that jacks are placed in various locations, for example, the kitchen, dinette, or living room. Since shopping by phone is recommended, you'll be spending a lot of time on the phone. Be sure there is a phone jack in the purest environment. The phone in your bedroom should be used with a jack so that you can remove the phone whenever you wish.

Telephone Wires. Years ago, telephone companies used a very tiny, thin wire (not exposed cloth wire, but wire hidden within the walls). By special request, and without any additional charge, the telephone company can wire your house with that kind of wire. This means a smaller amount of exposure for you to tolerate.

Termite Control. Since most builders automatically treat the ground with chlordane before laying the foundation, it is necessary to specify in the contract that termite shields must be used instead of chlordane or any other chemical.

Toilet Seats. Make sure they are not made of plastic. Builders frequently use plastic instead of wood. Also, metal attachments are best for toilet paper. Wood is also all right—anything but plastic.

Trash Compacters. We do not recommend trash compacters. It is too easy to put things in and leave them there for several days because it appears there is not much in the compacter. There is then the danger of mold growth. Besides, it produces an odor that can linger on.

Vacuum. Central vacuum systems with metal ducts work well. They should be vented outside. The motor can be placed in the basement. For the dust-sensitive person, Rex Air, which traps dust in the water, is the most satisfactory portable vacuum cleaner we have found. Other vacuum cleaners blow the dust around, and motor oil causes fumes that are objectionable to allergic sufferers.

Venetian Blinds. Even if you could get 100 percent metal Venetian blinds without any plastic parts, they are not advisable. They are dust collectors.

Ventilation. At the time that you are building your house, it is not much of an added expense to install several large fans. If you can afford it, it is recommended for every floor in your house. Even an unfinished basement should have a large fan for two reasons: (1) It is not so likely that mold will form when there is good ventilation, and (2) whenever there are bad fumes, the house can be cleared more quickly if there are several fans going.

One woman said she considered fans the best investment she had ever made. If someone comes into her house and lights a cigarette before she can stop him, or if a guest is heavily perfumed, she can more quickly remove the toxins from the air. Also, when she is reacting, she frequently forgets to turn off her stove. If the food and the pots burn, smoke permeates the house, and it takes less time to clear out the smoke with fans.

Wall Covering. An ideal wall covering for a sensitive person is one that is completely inert such as ceramic tile, which comes in attractive patterns, 4″ × 4″. Porcelain steel is good, too.

Wallpaper and Paste. Beware of vinyl wallpaper. However, those who can tolerate aluminum can find beautiful aluminum wallpaper. Just be sure there is no Mylar in it. You can apply it with Elmer's paste or wheat paste that you make or buy. Don't use wheat paste if you are sensitive to wheat.

Walls. Plaster walls, textured and colored and without paint, are best. Try nonasbestos wallboard. Plaster browncoat is unfibered gypsum and sand; browncoat is available (not deer hair, nylon and wood fibers). The unfibered type is recommended by the Bureau of Standards. Sand can be used in place of perlite. Dry wall is not good because of its glue content and other toxins.

Wall Switches. Unless you request otherwise, the plates that surround your light switches and your electric plugs, will be plastic. The difference in the cost is about eleven to fifteen cents per plate for metal. If expense is no object, ceramic plates are even more attractive.

Wall Vacuum. Don't let anyone talk you out of centralized vacuuming. At the time you are building your house the cost is not much more than buying the kind of vacuum that has to go through water. One patient reported that she neglected doing so because she was afraid the parts that were plastic would smell too strong. After two years, however, she found out that those plastics did not bother her so much as the plastic parts of her portable cleaner. When the vacuum is centralized, the dust does not come back into the air.

Water Filter. Dr. Theron Randolph recommends the use of the Puro Water Filter.[2] This rental unit has been installed in the homes of well over fifty of his allergic patients, and has proven satisfactory. Other filters, working on a similar principle, may be effective, but the effectiveness of one type has not been compared with another. "Since the Puro filter in the geographic area seems to answer the problem and the service has been satisfactory," he says, "I have merely continued to use and recommend it."

He points out that the majority of patients seemed to be helped either by filtration which removes chlorine or by boiling city water supplies, and that therefore it would appear that "chlorination of the water is at least one of the sources of difficulty, if not the most common source. It also appears that chlorination is the largest single factor in municipal water supplies which causes reactions. . . .

"One of the drawbacks in the use of the Puro filter is the fact that this rental service is not available in all localities. The company however, is making efforts to distribute these filters to persons not ordinarily serviced."

Waterproofing. Thoro-seal, manufactured by Standard Dry Wall Products, Inc., has in the past been used safely by some people.

Water Repellent. The water repellent that seems to work well is Euclid Integral. Although a chemical compound, Euclid is considered to be less objectionable than tar. Sta-Dri loses its toxicity in a few days and has been satisfactory for some.

Well Water. If you intend to have well water, be sure to have the water tested before you go to the expense of putting in the well. In some areas, there is so much detergent in well water, it is not safe to drink. In other areas, the mineral content is bad. If you decide to have city water instead, also have it checked for purity. Do not line wells or pipes with plastic. Use galvanized pipes.

Windows. Untreated wood can be obtained at no additional cost through B & B Wood Products Co., of Bedford Heights, Ohio. Aluminum might be a better choice if stains and finishes cannot be used. Use Thermopane windows in lieu of storm windows to avoid vinyl glue.

Wiring. BX cable is most easily tolerated. Check plastic-insulated types for odor. If asked, the telephone company can supply special wire; their regular wire is plasticized.

CHAPTER 24

Cleaning

B EFORE YOU go overboard with any new product to be used in large areas of your home, first test it on a small surface to see your reaction. One man we know who didn't, paid for it. He purchased a house that seemed quite compatible to him. Because there were so many untreated hardwood floors, he decided to use a varnish on them that was considered fairly nontoxic. It was labeled safe to use.

After the family moved in, he found that the only room in the house where he could be comfortable was a large tiled bathroom. Because the varnished floors were so troublesome, he had to live away from home for several months.

This does not suggest that for prevention purposes all varnishes and floor finishes should be avoided. It does mean to convey the idea that these products are pollutants in the home. When you choose any substance, it is suggested that you try it on a small piece of wood or material that you are going to be using. Place the sample on your pillow and sleep with it there overnight. If you can smell it or if you have a bad night's rest, it may be too toxic for you to use whether or not you have an allergy problem.

There are so many dangerously toxic products on the market that everyone, chemically sensitive or not, is well advised to use caution. Newspaper articles about the dangers of aerosol cans cause one to wonder why anyone would use them.

This chapter outlines methods of cleaning, using the greatest precautions for extreme cases of sensitivity and recommending products that seem to be the least offensive. It may be of interest that readers report they are surprised that many of these products are more effective than the toxic substances.

Before using any cleaning aid, test it in small quantities. Some things purchased and later found not tolerable can always be sold or given away. However, if it has been used on a large surface (like the floors), you may find that the offending odor can never be totally eliminated.

Remember: *No product is safe for everyone.*

HOUSEHOLD CLEANING AIDS

All-purpose Baking Soda. Baking soda quickly removes stale odors. It is ideal for freshening both the inside and outside of refrigerators, freezers, breadboxes, canisters, and lunch boxes. Mix three tablespoons of baking soda with 1 quart of water to make the freshening solution. The same mixture can be used for cleaning a variety of things, such as stainless steel surfaces and even a baby's diaper pail.

Coffeemakers and teapots frequently need a thorough "freshening" to remove oils and stains that collect on the sides. Baking soda can come to the rescue for all nonaluminum materials. Use it as a cleanser poured on a damp sponge, or in the case of a percolator, add three tablespoons of baking soda to a full pot of water and let the coffeemaker run through the complete perking cycle.

Working with foods such as onions, garlic, and fish leaves unpleasant odors on hands. Wash hands with baking soda. The results are very effective.

Soda makes an excellent fire extinguisher for kitchen grease fires. Throw it on the fire to suffocate the flames. Keep a box in the family car to extinguish engine fires. It will not harm the engine. Throw the baking soda on the flames, and to prevent the flames from flying back, be sure to throw the soda *with* the wind.

Sprinkle baking soda on a damp sponge to wash away bugs and road grease from windshields, windshield wipers, and headlights. Use it the same way for cleaning chrome, sinks, tubs.

Grease stains on car and household rugs can be removed with baking soda which absorbs the grease. Rub the soda into the spot with a cloth or brush; then sweep away the residue.

The list of items that can be cleaned and freshened with baking soda includes ashtrays, babies' rubber pants, the sole-plate of irons, thermos bottles, casseroles, ice-cube trays, vases, combs and brushes, a pet's dishes, and even your teeth.

All-purpose Cleaners. Use baking soda as a substitute for scouring powders. Salt water or vinegar and water can be used as all-purpose cleaners, too. For example, shower stalls can be washed with the solution to cut the soap film that breaks down the grouting, and it leaves a high gloss on the tile. Vinegar and water add a gleam to windows, and make stainless steel sparkle. Vinegar is effective against mold. Salt water is effective on Formica, glass, marble, and metals.

Cleaning Agents. Borax is an effective, nontoxic cleaning agent. It was found to be an effective disinfectant in the ecologic unit of a hospital where 20-Mule Team borax was used. Use it in your daily washing and cleaning after you have tested it to see if you are sensitive to it.

As a scouring powder poured on a damp sponge, borax is effective on porcelain tubs and sinks, Formica counter tops, bathroom tile, and stainless steel sinks and appliances.

Oakite is a good heavy-duty cleaning agent (tri-sodium phosphate). Oakite has been found to be safe for many sensitive persons, and is useful as a general cleaning compound.[1]

Tri-Sodium Phosphate (TSP). If Oakite is not available, you may be able to use tri-sodium phosphate as a substitute. Test carefully for sensitivity. Tri-sodium phosphate is an effective cleaning compound used by some allergic persons for surface cleaning. Precaution should be taken against absorption through the skin by wearing cotton-lined "Bluette" rubber gloves. TSP may be purchased by the pound through your hardware stores. Experiment with a quarter cup per two gallons warm water and either increase or decrease as desired. It works miracles with fingerprints on painted walls and woodwork. TSP is poisonous if swallowed, so *clearly label and store away from children.*

Zephiran in water is useful as an antibacterial skin cleanser, and is also effective as a disinfectant, especially as an antimold disinfectant. It can be used to wipe walls and floors of basements.

HOUSEHOLD TIPS

Brass. Lemon juice or vinegar with salt cleans brass and steel.

Brushes. To clean dried paint brushes, simmer them for ten minutes in a pint of vinegar.

Charcoal. Activated charcoal absorbs odors in closets, basements, storerooms, rooms with motors, and in refrigerators.

Chrome. Use a soft dry cloth dipped in pure cider vinegar to wipe chrome clean.

Cleaning Brushes. Wooden-handled, natural bristle brushes are manufactured by the Quickee Manufacturing Corp. of Philadelphia, Pennsylvania: Bowl Brush #B302, Bottle Brush #K203, Tampico Vegetable Brush #K202, Scrub (Sink) Brush #104. Wash all new items well before using.

Dishwasher. For periodic cleaning, put 1 cup vinegar into the empty dishwasher and run it through the cycle.

Drains. A handful of baking soda plus a half glass of vinegar poured down a drainpipe and covered tightly for a minute will open a stopped-up drain.

To keep drains from clogging, use three tablespoons sal soda (washing soda) once or twice a week. Note: At least one plumber we know of prefers this since he does not have to protect himself from fumes and skin contact; he claims it is just as effective as the commercial chemical formulas.

Dust. It is suggested that anyone with an extreme dust sensitivity wear a dampened cotton surgical mask when doing work that stirs up dust particles.

Flea Control. Grind banana peel and place in strategic spots in home to combat fleas from pets. Sprinkle rock salt on rug, leave a few days, and vacuum.

Floor. Floor finish: Spenser Kellogg pure raw linseed oil, half oil and vinegar solution. Apply in thin coat. Rub in well. Dries in four days. Suggest nonelectric floor polisher. Warning: Some people are very sensitive to linseed.

Furniture. Mayonnaise may be used to polish furniture. *Raw*, not boiled, linseed can be a very effective cleaner. Consider using beeswax and oil in combination. Sensitive patients, test with caution. An oiled wood finish on furniture can be maintained by rubbing olive or lemon oil into the wood and leather. Other oils such as vegetable and nut oils can be used, but they have a tendency to turn rancid.

Furniture Care. To renovate leather furniture, use a solution of 1 cup vinegar with 1 cup linseed oil. See Wax Buildup for additional hints. Sensitive patients, test with caution.

Grease. A paste of Fuller's Earth and Water applied to electric burners absorbs residual grease. Rinse. This same paste can be applied to a grease spot on wallpaper; let dry and brush off. If you are sensitive to Fuller's Earth and Water, substitute baking soda.

Gum. To remove chewing gum from skin or carpeting, try applying Basic H, full strength.

Irons. To remove dark or burned spots from your electric iron, rub with heated vinegar and salt.

Mildew. To prevent black mildew from forming on door of refrigerator, wipe vinegar on the rubber cushion.

Mold Cleaning. Use Zephiran chloride, aqueous solution. Buy the concentrate, labeled 17 percent. Dilute one ounce with one gallon of water, or one unit (as one cc, or one tablespoon, to twenty-seven units of water). This is effective in cleaning showers, toilets, bathrooms, floors. Be sure that you put a liberal amount in the corners. The cleaning of moldy areas should not be done by anyone who is extremely sensitive to molds. Someone else in the family should take care of this.

Borax in water is another good mold retardant. Of course, the best way to manage mold, is to prevent it wherever possible. Keep dry cloths available in the bathroom so that shower, tub, basin, and floor can be wiped dry after each use. The cloths along with wet towels and washcloth should then be hung to dry in a basement area.

Never place slightly damp clothes in a closet or in a drawer. Once you have tried on an article of clothing or worn it for even a short period of time, do not put it back into your closet with clean clothes. One woman, highly sensitive to mold, found that the only way her closets remained free of mold was by leaving on a small light in the closet at all times. The heat from the light helped to retard the growth of mold.

Mothproofing. Salt sprinkled on rugs and furniture wards off moths.

Oven Cleaning. While the oven is still warm wipe with a damp cloth. Soak racks in a solution of Amway LOC in very hot water. Washing soda and steel wool can be used. Quick Glo Oven Cleaner is said to be nontoxic and fume free; it also cleans aluminum windows. It is available in some department stores.

To clean a broiler grill or oven bottom where food has spilled, sprinkle with Bon Ami cleanser while still hot, cover with absorbent towels and sprinkle with water. Most of the soil will be absorbed by steam and towels.

Pesticides. Do not use Shell Pest Strip as it contains toxic chemicals. Good sanitation, storage, lighting, mouse traps, and fly swatters are effective measures against pests.

Pipes. Equal parts of salt and baking soda can clear pipes of clogged soap and scum.

Pots and Pans. Soaking in salt water is an effective method for removing food which has adhered to pots and pans.

Refrigerator. Leave an open box of baking soda in the refrigerator for deodorizing. Replace in three months. Pour the old box down the drain to deodorize.

Rugs. Clean rugs with cabbage. Cut cabbage head in half, rub into the rug with the cut side down. As edges soil, cut off and continue to use. Vacuum thoroughly to remove all particles of the cabbage. Restore faded rugs by rubbing a strong salt-water solution into the rug with a damp cloth.

Soap. Soaps best tolerated, are, in this order: Rokeach kosher soap, Ivory soap, Bon Ami cake soap. (Rokeach, a coconut oil soap, seems easiest on the hands.) For washing dishes use Ivory or Rokeach soap with plain steel wool. To remove grease, use Bon Ami cake soap or baking soda.

Because it is so difficult to find a pure soap in a powder or flake form, some people have to make up a form of liquid soap that will work in a washing machine.

Use three bars of a pure soap you can tolerate, whether it be Rokeach's, Ivory, or a face soap. Place them in a glass jar, fill with water and soak for three or four days or even longer if possible. When the soap is soft enough, place it in a blender with additional water and blend until smooth. If you have a crock pot, you can speed up the process, by placing the soft soap covered with a large quantity of water in the pot, and let it cook on low until it is totally melted. Pour the liquid into Mason jars and let stand. Within a day or two, some of it will solidify, but it melts quickly in a pan of water on low heat.

To launder clothes let hot water pour into the washing machine to mix with the liquid soap. Then proceed in your customary way. For those who are so sensitive that even a mild soap like Ivory or Rokeach's is troublesome, try washing a few garments with this liquid soap, rinse with vinegar, then rinse again with plain cold water.

For pots and pans and general housecleaning requiring an abrasive cleaning agent, grate Bon Ami cake soap. Store in a glass Mason jar. Use as any other cleanser. Very effective with Supreme brand steel wool. Supreme contains no soap or detergent.

Silver. Sterling silver can be cleaned with a soupy solution of baking soda and water, or with cream of tartar plus water in an aluminum pan or aluminum foil. To be effective, the silver must touch the aluminum.

Stainless Steel. Use vinegar to clean spots from stainless steel kitchen equipment.

Steel Wool. Supreme brand, soaped thoroughly makes an effective cleaner. Because it disintegrates easily and can cause infections, do not soak in water, tear apart, or use more than once. Rokeach steel wool soap pads have also been tolerated by some sensitive people.

Vinegar. In general, vinegar, salt, and baking soda are excellent deodorizers and cleaners. When you have a cleaning problem, try them before you try anything else.

Washing Machine. Salt added to the washing machine helps to prevent colors from running. Twice a year use one gallon of distilled vinegar in an empty washing machine or dishwasher to increase the efficiency of your machine. Remember that front-loading washing machines use less water and soap.

Wax Buildup. For a simple case of wax buildup, three tablespoons of sal soda to a quart of water sponged over the surface, rinsed with fresh water and wiped dry, is the prescribed "cure." For varnish, lacquer, or shellac, use a cup of sal soda to a quart of water and apply the solution to one small area at a time with medium steel wool. Rinse, wipe dry. Run over the surface lightly with fine sandpaper. Wrap sandpaper around a block of wood for table surfaces, and around a hard dry cellulose sponge for chairs. The sponge has just enough give to let the sandpaper dig into the rounded and fluted areas. Be sure the wood is completely dry before applying desired finish.

Windows. To clean, use solution of one tablespoon of vinegar to one to two quarts water. To remove paint from windows, heat vinegar and apply. To clean mirrors or windows, saturate wet cloth, rub with Bon Ami cake soap, and apply to glass. Rinse off with clear cold water and dry with absorbent toweling.

TIPS FOR CLEANING CLOTHES

Bleach. Whitener for clothes: Miracle White, available at supermarkets, is nontoxic and biodegradable. Not good for the extremely sensitive patient. Borax is a natural bleach and mold retardant. Sprinkled in mold-producing places, it acts as a deodorant. Used for laundering, it is an effective whitener.

Boots. To remove white stains on boots after winter snows, apply a solution of vinegar and water to a clean cloth and rub lightly.

Detergents. Avoid detergents, especially those made with perfumes, softeners, phosphorous or enzymes. Instead, use soap, vinegar, baking soda, borax or a combination of these.

A woman, allergic to many laundry products, finally resorted to washing her clothes in baking soda, a product she could tolerate. Unfortunately, she did not know how to prevent her clothes from developing a gray look.

A friend offered to wash these clothes with a brightening detergent and promised to rinse carefully with vinegar and then clear water. The uninformed friend used a detergent with enzymes. Enzymes never rinse out. As a result all the detergent-laundered items were useless to the allergic woman.

Dry Cleaners. Locate a dry cleaner in your community who will use the old-fashioned petroleum cleaner and omit mothproofing treatment. Extremely sensitive patients should avoid dry cleaning entirely, if possible. Some with severe allergies cannot tolerate petroleum cleaner at all, but others find that airing clothes after dry cleaning is helpful. One patient, however, had to air her clothes for three weeks before she could wear them.

Naphtha, a petroleum solvent—*not* perchlorethylene—is recommended for dry cleaning. Be sure the dry cleaner uses distilled naphtha without added detergents. You may have to send a large amount of clothing to your dry cleaner at one time to make it worth his while to follow your directions. Thus it might be advisable to organize a group to send clothes to the same dry cleaner together.

Stains. For stains on cotton or linen clothing, wet with lemon juice, sprinkle with salt, and place in the sun. To remove scorch marks from cottons, saturate area with vinegar and wash as usual.

Washing Clothes. When washing clothes, use ½ cup of vinegar in rinse water to neutralize the odor of the cleaning agent. Dr. Alsoph Corwin, a biochemist, suggests that Alconox be used in the washing machine to inhibit mold formation. Molds grow better in cotton and kapok than in wool, he says, because they contain the enzyme cellulase. He has also found that salt and especially perspiration greatly enhance mold growth. Those highly sensitive to molds should wash pillow cases, sheets, and sleepwear after each night's use, and should never hang cotton clothes back in the closet after they have been worn. A freshly laundered shirt keeps quite well in the closet, but molds form on a used one within twenty-four hours.

CHAPTER 25

Pest Control: Insects and Rodents

INSECTS and rodents are part of our world and a problem that must be faced without hysteria. Don't press the panic button and rush to buy harmful chemicals. It is not necessary to pollute your environment in order to get rid of these unwelcome guests. Here are suggestions to combat the problem rationally and without detriment to allergic persons.*

RODENTS

Mice

Mice usually come into homes out of surrounding fields and yards every fall, and require some action on the part of the home owner at that time. The small snap traps baited with cheese, bacon, or chocolate can usually be used successfully to catch them. Several other types of traps are also available, including small size Hav-a-Heart catch-'em-alive ones. Traps, preferred to poison, avoid the risk of an odor resulting from the mice crawling off to die.

As with roaches, cleanliness is important. To shut off food supplies, alternate the bait for the trap or poison you supply. If you drop one crumb, pick it up. Even more important is bait attractiveness. If the bait can be more attractive than any other food around, it is possible to clean up rodent pests, even in a feed mill or restaurant with a great deal of other food around. If the mice get bait-shy, the bait should be changed.

If possible, try to locate the points of entry of the mice and plug them with steel wool.

Various baits such as De-Con and Zurd poisoned with warfarin are commercially available. These often work quite well. Sometimes Harris roach tablets work for mice. One's own baits can also be prepared using

* For the material in this chapter, the authors are deeply indebted to Francis Silver, P.E., a registered chemical and environmental engineer whose work is presented here almost in its entirety.

214

fresh ground cornmeal, 10 to 20 parts to 1 part of warfarin. Flour to which has been added a little sugar and cocoa and about 25 percent to 50 percent plaster of paris can be used and offers little hazard to children or pets.

Great care should be taken to see that mice do not get into furniture, especially of the overstuffed variety. If mice are around, check furniture frequently to be sure that there are no holes in it. Close up any holes with tape, tacks, or other method.

Mice, like roaches, are basically a tenant's responsibility rather than a landlord's.

Rats

An important part of any rat control effort is to fill in their holes and break up their nests as often as required up to several times a week. Rat-proofing of buildings by closing up all points of entry is also important.

Several kinds of poisoned baits and traps can be used. These can be placed in boxes with holes big enough to admit the rat but keep out birds and cats. For several decades warfarin has been the rat poison of choice because it is slow acting and less likely to arouse bait-shyness. Baits can be made more attractive by adding bacon grease to cereal baits like corn, wheat, or oats but this may make the bait more attractive to cats and requires more care in placement. Ten pounds of fresh-ground corn meal to which has been added one pound of dry powdered warfarin has been used by farmers to kill rats in corn cribs. The aroma and convenience of the fresh-ground corn meal is so attractive to the rats that they will eat it to their death in preference to eating the corn off the cob.

Rats like holes. A board placed on the ground on its edge and leaned against a wall creates a tunnel into which snap traps or poisoned baits can be placed. Rats will like to run through it, and even if they do not eat the bait on the trap, just running over it may catch them.

People who use cats to curb rats must take good care of and feed the cats so they will be strong enough to fight the rats. They must not expect the cats to live off the rats. Ferrets and fumigation are also used in rat control, but these are usually beyond the scope of amateurs.

Either landlord or tenant could assume responsibility for rat control, or better still, both can work together on the problem. Certainly neither can claim irresponsibility. The newspaper reporters, social workers, and tenants who blame all roach, mouse, and rat problems on landlords have done a great deal to perpetuate these problems by encouraging tenant irresponsibility.

INSECTS

Description	Habits	Possible Control Methods	Unacceptable Control Methods Inside Buildings Because of Human Toxicity
Ants Large or small, black, red, or half and half. Large black carpenter ants.	Food left around brings them. Many like sweet food. Others prefer grease.	1. Cleanliness; no crumbs left around, clean sink. 2. Red Pepper. 3. Mint planted by the front and back door of a house has prevented ants from entering. 4. Borax or boric acid.	Any war-gas type of insecticide painted, sprayed, squirted, or vaporized by tenant, home owner, pest control operator, or landlord. Pyrethrum, rotenone.
Beetles		1. Keep insect (sawtoothed grain beetle) out of cereals, cracker meal, cookies, flour, and macaroni by placing a bay leaf in each container.	
Moths *Clothes Moth* Tiny moth about half as big as cereal moth. Other stage is small white worm that eats woolens, hair, fur, natural bristles, leaving some webbing or cocoons.	Likes dark, quiet, still locations. Soft-bodied. Cannot stand light activity. Avoids light, sun, air. Cannot live in blankets on bed that is slept in once a week or on a suit worn once a week. Does not require water.	1. Use mechanical methods rather than chemical. Keep clothes out in light and move occasionally. 2. Good stiff brushing will kill eggs, larvae and other forms. 3. Wrap in newsprint or brown wrapping paper. Seal in paper bags or in zipper bags. (Be certain clothes are clean first. Use masking tape to seal up small holes.)	Paradichlorobenzene, napthalene moth balls, moth flakes, moth nuggets, moth crystals, peach gas, camphor (except in a closet, large garbage can, or other fumigating chamber, *outside the house*). Moth proofing sprays using chloropicrin, paradichlorobenzene, dieldrin, or other volatile insecticides.

Carpet Beetle
or
Buffalo Beetle

Grayish round-backed beetle shaped like a lady bug but about half the size. Some varieties are oval rather than round, and black rather than gray.

Habits similar to clothes moth above. Can live on lint or linty dust, toe nails, horn, or other keratin. Does not require water. Likes wool soiled with food spilled in the lap or urine in crotch of trousers, so eats there first. Can be brought in from store or dry cleaners.

4. Wear once a week in season and then have cleaned. When returned check and then seal openings in bag with masking tape.
5. Dried tobacco plant in closet or chest.
6. Pepper corns in a chest.
7. Lavender.
8. Vacuum rugs, hang on line outside and beat with a rug beater.
9. Store in a chest, closet, or fumigating chamber outside the house.
10. Some limited use of mineral type of insecticides such as silcofluorides might be acceptable for top coats or other items not in direct contact with skin for nonsensitive persons. These ruin the feel of furs, cashmeres, vicuna, and should not be used on them.
11. Heat or cold fumigation. Air from time to time in the sun or wrap in paper and put into your freezer for 3 to 7 days.
12. Washing or dry cleaning kills all forms.

217

INSECTS (cont.)

Description	Habits	Possible Control Methods	Unacceptable Control Methods Inside Buildings Because of Human Toxicity
Fleas Small (⅛″) jumping, brown insect that is so hard that it is extremely difficult to crush.	Feeds on blood of dogs, cats, mules, horses. Bites certain people but not everyone.	1. Catch and kill them between thumbnail and finger nail. 2. Probably a little squirt of solvent or gasoline on a dog might kill them. 3. A few 2′ squares of roofing on which has been placed a tablespoonful of creosote has worked for a terrible infestation after dogs left a house. People did not stay in building for week that creosote was there. 4. Eucalyptus, leaves or perhaps oil, has been known to keep fleas off pets. 5. Feed your pet with Brewers Yeast. If your pet will eat it, the powder form in his food is preferred. Otherwise use pill form, as many as your pet will take.	Painting on or spraying or squirting of war-gas type of insecticides, Raid, pyrethrum, rotenone; flea collar containing lindane or other war-gas type insecticide. Systemic insecticide fed to dog (if you value the animal).

Flies, House Flies, Cluster Flies

Everybody knows what a fly looks like. May be black, greenish, gray.

Lays eggs in rotten flesh, dung, manure, decaying vegetable matter, earthworms, garbage. These hatch into maggots and later turn into flies.

1. Vacuum cleaner for cluster flies in attic.
2. Fly ribbons.
3. Fly paper laid on decorative fixture near ceiling.
4. Window and door screens.
5. Fly swatter.
6. Flies alighting on a window or door screen usually walk up, not down. If the top 4″ of the screen is cut out and another piece of screen put inside to lap over the lower section about an inch or two, but gapped about ¼″, this forms a kind of check valve that lets the flies walk up and outside the building.
7. Electrocutors for outdoor fly problems and some indoor ones.
8. Fly trap made of screen wire using funnel and bait at bottom.
9. Garbage should be covered, ground, or enclosed in bags. Manure should be composted.
10. Purple martins outside.

Fogging with insecticide, No-Pest Strips except outside in garbage can or catch basin, lindane or DDT vaporizers, aerosol bombs, sprays, Raid, paint-on insecticides, pyrethrum, rotenone, time-mist dispenser.

INSECTS (cont.)

Description	Habits	Possible Control Methods	Unacceptable Control Methods Inside Buildings Because of Human Toxicity
Mosquitoes A small insect that flies about at night and bites people.	Less active during day. Lays eggs in water which hatch later.	1. Screens. 2. Kill them on the window screens at daybreak. 3. Suck them into the vacuum cleaner at night off the ceiling using the long "wand." 4. Try to destroy their breeding places by emptying tin cans, old tires, clogged or improperly sloped spouting. 5. Purple martins and other insect catching birds. 6. Oil on breeding water. One of the oil or chemical companies has developed a new compound that is supposed to be much better than oil. 7. Electrocutors.	Spraying, vaporizing, or fogging insecticides into the air.

Cereal Moth, Weevil, Cigarette or Drugstore Beetles

The confused beetle or weevil is about ⅛″ to 3/16″ long. It is elongated oval in shape. Reddish brown in color.

The cereal moth is a small, grayish, moth, about twice as big as a clothes moth. It eats in the larval stage.

Drugstore and cigarette beetles are small, brown, flying beetles. They are several times as large as a flea.

All of these insects infest grain and cereal products.

1. Do a thorough housekeeping job on the kitchen to find out where they are coming from. Throw out all contaminated cereal products.
2. Fly ribbons hung inside the shade of a floor lamp have been found to aid greatly in control of an infestation of drugstore beetles from Milk Bone crackers for dogs.
3. Kill all you see.
4. Clean cracks in kitchen where food has built up.
5. Freeze flours and grains for at least 48 to 72 hours. Then, if freezer space is a problem, store in tightly sealed glass jars in the coolest place in the house.

Spraying, fogging, painting-on, squirting war-gas type of insecticides. Vaporizers.

INSECTS (cont.)

Description	Habits	Possible Control Methods	Unacceptable Control Methods Inside Buildings Because of Human Toxicity
German or Small Kitchen Roach Reddish brown to yellowish brown. Elongated oval shape. About ¾" long when fully grown. Females may drag egg cases behind them. Fast-moving.	Loves dampness, mildew, mustiness, water. Stays out of sight in cracks until room is dark and then appears.	1. Meticulous cleanliness, no crumbs on floor. The scorched earth policy of nothing for them to eat; no garbage left around very long, no food out, no dirty dishes in sink. Discard bags and boxes brought in from grocery. 2. Boric acid sprinkled liberally in crevices, corners, nesting places, around the molding. They will disappear in about 6 weeks. Then, keep the worst areas sparsely covered with boric acid. 3. Sodium fluoride powder sprinkled around behind stove, refrigerator, in cracks, in kitchen and wherever there is water. An excellent remedy, rather safe because a low volatile mineral even though quite toxic if stirred	Poisoned food item, like doughnut. Too inviting to children or pets. Spraying or squirting, volatile, post-World War II insecticides around by building management or pest control service. (This gives off toxic fumes and is not most effective.) Raid, Real-Kill, Hot Shot, No-Roach, No-Pest Strip, Lindane Vaporizer, (either one shot or continuous), clock-operated pyrethrum or other insecticide dispenser (time-mist). Fogging with insecticide, pyrethrum, rotenone, Chlordane, Malathion, Diazinon, Baygon, Sevin, Parathion. *Important:* Put any poisoned bait out of reach of pets or children, behind stove or refrigerator.

up and breathed. Hard to find since about 1970 as taken off market by government.

4. Japanese roach trap. An actual trap door trap of plastic and metal. Bait with banana, etc.

5. Turn lights on at night and step on roaches or use an old dinner knife to kill all you can see, especially in cracks.

6. Make your own roach powder: Mix 2 tbsp. flour, 1 tbsp. cocoa powder and 4 tbsp. powdered borax. Store in plainly labeled glass container. To use, sprinkle mixture on small pieces of paper and place where roaches have been seen.

7. Cucumber rinds.

8. Roach hives or tubes.

9. Box turtle.

INSECTS (cont.)

Description	Habits	Possible Control Methods	Unacceptable Control Methods Inside Buildings Because of Human Toxicity
Big Roaches: American Roach or Palmetto Bug Reddish brown to yellowish brown color, long oval shape, about 2" long when fully grown.	Loves dampness, mildew, mustiness, water; stays out of sight in cracks until room is dark and then appears. Lives in sewer.	1. Harris roach tablet is a specific for them. Put under or behind things so children or pets cannot get. 2. Fill traps into sewer with water or seal off floor drain with heavy metal plate or tin. 3. Look around inside and outside to see where they might be coming from (septic tank, sewer, cess pool, privy, etc.). 4. Japanese roach trap baited with banana. 5. Make your own trap out of quart Mason jar set upright, no top, grease inside of neck. Bait with banana. Place flat stick against side as a walkway, up and in. 6. Sodium fluoride, borax, boric acid. 7. Make your own concoction. 8. Cucumber rinds.	Insecticide vaporizers or foggers. War-gas type insecticides sprayed, dusted, squirted, or painted on. Pyrethrum, rotenone, DDT (see German roach for more details).

Oriental Roach—Black Water Bug

Glossy black, as wide as long. About as big as a thumbnail.

Can live and multiply on dog dung.

1. See German roach.

Silver Fish and Fire Brats

About ½" long, cream or tan or brown, silvery, soft-bodied, fast-moving, then motionless.

Can live outside in leaves and grass and so constantly invade house. Paper and starch sizing on paper and starch sizing on paper are favorite foods. Sometimes eat fabrics. They live about 2 years. Lay one or two hundred eggs.

1. Vacuum cleaner.
2. Trap made of empty cold cream jar; no top; strip of adhesive tape up outside so bug can climb up; ½ tsp. of flour inside for bait.
3. 5 or 10% boric acid or sodium fluoride and 90% flour. Some powdered sugar could be added. Put around where they are.
4. Cats kill them.
5. Kill every one you see.
6. Regular heavy housecleaning once or twice a year to break up their abode and kill most of them.

See German roach.

War-gas type of insecticides sprayed, squirted, painted-on, fogged, or vaporized. Raid, Real-Kill, etc.

Spider Mites

1. Fresh banana peels in infested areas. Until the infestation has cleared, keep adding fresh peels to the dried ones.
2. Make mixture of: 4 cups wheat flour, ½ cup buttermilk, 5 gal. water. Spray on ornamental plants to rid of mites.

225

INSECTS (cont.)

Description	Habits	Possible Control Methods	Unacceptable Control Methods Inside Buildings Because of Human Toxicity
Termites Appearance similar to ant, but brownish color instead of red or black, and no wasp waist such as ant has.	Winged ones swarm in spring around April. Subterranean variety most common, must return to earth to get water every 24 hours; dampness attracts them. (Dry wood termite does not require water.) Rare in northern latitudes. Become increasingly virulent in tropical climates, much less common in cold climates.	1. Do not panic and rush into war-gas treatment that makes your house uninhabitable. They do not eat fast in northern latitudes. Simply breaking tubes has been known to destroy them. Sometimes they just die out. High water table in ground may drown nest. 2. Build termite shields; must be lock seamed, or large lap, and stick out at least 1½″ to 2″ inside and outside. Ground level around house must be at least 6″ below termite shield, 18″ below top of finished floor. Do not try to avoid that step or two up; it can cost you your house or your health if you do. If they are already in the house, have a good, honest and knowledgeable carpenter or mason tear out portion of wall and build them out (not using volatile insecticides).	Chlordane or other volatile insecticides. Do not treat ground under slab with volatile insecticides. Do not treat ground at all if you have your own well. Termites are bad but poisoning your water or the air in your house is worse.

3. Heat. Fumigate small infestations (120° F. for 10 hours or 140° F. for 10 minutes will kill all insect life) using heat lamp.
4. Experiment with baited poison such as ant trap.
5. A sheet of copper 18" wide around outside of foundation, inserted 1' in ground has been reported to control them.
6. Copper chromate or cryolite or other nonvolatile insecticide such as was used before war-gas insecticides by pest control operator.
7. Dryness.

Ticks, Brown Dog Ticks

Oval, looks like a crab. Moves very slowly. 8 legs when mature. Brownish. ⅛" to ¼" across. After filling with blood, about the size of a small raspberry.

Ticks love to get on back of neck in hairline, but can be anywhere. Apparently they can move on the human body without being felt.

1. Put gasoline in a small oil can. (Solvent might do but have not tested it. Alcohol will not do.) Examine dog once a day, preferably in afternoon or evening and put drop of gasoline on each tick found. This will kill tick and they will drop off and die. In a few weeks this process will get rid of all ticks in neighborhood where dog roams.

Pulling ticks off with pliers. (It usually pulls a piece of flesh with the tick and dog soon avoids you.) Burning tick with a match can be a fire hazard, usually does not work too well. Spraying dog with Malathion or other war-gas type of chemical. Flea collars. Feeding a systemic insecticide to dog that poisons tick when it bites dog. (Likely to affect dog's health adversely in time.)

Unlike the currently used roach-control methods of most exterminators (which are unacceptable safety-wise), their methods for rat control are usually effective and acceptable by safety standards. However, usually tenants or landlords by themselves or cooperatively can learn to do an effective job if they will study the problem and work aggressively at controlling it. What they lack in skill is, to a considerable extent, compensated for by the fact that they are there so much of the time instead of just once or twice a month. The sense of accomplishment and feeling of independence that comes from mastering a pest problem yourself can be very rewarding and easily worth the trouble.

CHAPTER 26

Choosing Clothing and Fabrics

THIS STORY of one person's problem and how he solved it may help you very much. (He gave permission to use his real name, Jim Sherry.)

Jim suffered from severe headaches, phlebitis, and other symptoms. His wife found him irritable and overtired. She worked in a hospital which had an ecology unit, and she had heard some weird stories about the unit and the doctor who prescribed "crazy meals." But his wife was desperate enough to suggest anything that would help her husband, no matter how far-fetched. The director of nurses with whom she talked gave her a glowing report of how people had been helped, and so Mrs. Sherry persuaded her husband to enter the unit. Jim Sherry was then found to be allergic to many things, including synthetics like polyester, Dacron, nylon, and even to the chemical treatment in some natural fabrics like cotton.

After eliminating the offending fabrics, the phlebitis disappeared except when Jim was exposed to something to which he is sensitive. He has had no headaches for a year-and-a-half. He is now playing tennis and softball for the first time in twenty-five years. He is a man forty-five years of age, "having a blast." It would have been too much for him to try these sports before, but now the change in him is so noticeable that his daughter keeps remarking, "Gee, Daddy's nice, pleasant to live with."

Although Jim is still under constant exposure to allergens, the change is quite obvious. Of course, during vacations where he can select a controlled environment, he is an absolute delight. His home has been cleared of all the pollutants that bother him. When he goes away for a three-day business trip, within a day after having been in a hotel with a carpet, his phlebitis is back. Fortunately, it clears up quickly after he returns to his clean environment.

This story is of particular interest for a special reason. Although Jim needs pure, natural fabrics, he found that he was having trouble getting them. There are years when cotton is plentiful, and years when you cannot get it easily. Even when cottons are plentiful, they are frequently contaminated with toxic materials to make them iron-free, wrinkle-free, or permanent-press. In addition, manufacturers have developed the very poor practice of combining natural fabrics with synthetic materials. Even in "cotton" towels 10 or 15 percent polyester or some other synthetic is often used.

Jim realized that there were many people who were even more sensitive than he, and they too needed pure, natural materials. He checked through hospital sources, through hospital suppliers, but discovered orders must be placed for huge quantities. Then he found a man who had a personal interest, and who would spend hours in research to make sure cottons were pure. With the help of a group of patients and an interested doctor, Jim and his wife began a cotton co-op called Ecologists Cotton Co-op.[1]

Even with the care the co-op takes, they frequently receive fabric that includes a small percentage of polyester, and which must be sent back. Because it is a co-op they do not stock material. It must be ordered in advance.

The Ecologists Cotton Co-op prices—including shipping costs—are usually less than local prices. Many extremely allergic people all over the country have found this co-op to be a life-saver.

Barrier cloth is one of the fabrics which can be ordered from the Co-op. In one of the ecologic units in Texas, Dr. Rea has found that some patients can tolerate offending mattresses, if they are covered and sealed in with a cover of barrier cloth. This is a finely woven surgical cloth of pure cotton and totally untreated. It is used in the hospital operating room and its close weave prevents bacteria from penetrating.

Since barrier cloth is pure, most people can tolerate it, but it is suggested that individuals test it before paying for or ordering a large quantity for mattress and pillow covers. It might be helpful, also, for patients who are very allergic to dust.

TESTS FOR UNTREATED FABRICS

The best way of testing materials is through your own sensory system. Many people are able to determine for themselves whether they are allergic to materials such as a piece of yard goods, a rug, or even an appliance such as a TV set.

Francis Silver, P.E., consulting environmental engineer, believes that some people have such a keen sense of smell that "they can detect indiscreet chemicalization of a product" with their noses. "Others," he said, "have learned by themselves how to detect harmful chemicalization by touching with the palm of their hand."

That Crawly Feeling. This brings us to "that crawly feeling," which

Silver feels can guide a person in knowing what to buy or live with and what to avoid. As he explains it, the method, basically, is this:

"The palm of the hand is placed first on a chemically uncontaminated surface, giving no unusual feeling. If it is then placed on a chemically contaminated surface, a slight 'crawly' feeling will be felt after a few seconds to a minute or two.

"Some persons do not get the 'crawly feeling' but may get more of a 'tingly' or perhaps a 'bad' feeling. It feels as if the surface is 'alive' and 'not right.'

"The hand should rest lightly on the surface under test. The proper pressure is about half of the weight of the hand. It should not be rubbed over the surface or pressed heavily. If you rub, that will activate nerve endings and drown out the crawly feeling, which is probably being generated by pain nerves.

"The intensity of the feeling will be roughly proportional to the level of contamination. If the hand is removed from the contaminated surface, for some time afterward a peculiar or 'not quite right' feeling will still be felt in the hand."

Silver maintains that by moving the hand, first to the control object that does not affect you, then to the object which is suspect, and then back again, a level of reaction can be determined.

He says that several samples can be compared. "It can be determined that Sample A is more contaminated than Sample B, but less contaminated than Sample C."

Always test objects for the crawly feeling before buying any kind of textile, pillow, bedding, towels, clothing, or even furniture.

The scientific name for the process of testing an object with one's body is called "organoleptic measurement" or measurement by the senses. Coffee, tea, and wine tasters are organoleptic measurers, as are those who test perfumes with their noses.

Silver believes that about 50 percent of the population can train themselves to use organoleptic measurement, using their noses, taste buds, or the feel of something that gives one that crawly feeling.

Remember, it is far better to keep a shabby old rug that is not chemically contaminated than to buy a pretty new one that is going to ruin your health with toxic chemicals. As Francis Silver points out, "Design carelessness in the introduction of a wide variety of new and old chemicals into manufacturing is bringing about a quiet crisis. Insufficient weight has been given to the toxicity of many of these chemicals and to their potential for impairment of health over the long term."

Your best defense against these harmful products may lie in your own hand.

Water Bubble. The water-bubble test applies only to cotton. A drop of water will readily soak into untreated cotton unless the cloth is barrier cloth or a primitive fabric, such as unbleached muslin or rough Mexican cotton. Primitive fabrics have a strong vegetable smell but these sizings usually wash out easily.

Carry with you an eye dropper in a small medicine bottle filled with water. Drop a bubble of water on the fabric; if the bubble soaks in, *probably* it is untreated. If the bubble stands up on top, it is likely to be treated. Never use the bubble test exclusively; it should always be supplemented by another method before you purchase a large amount of the fabric.

Crush Test. Crush 100 percent cotton in your hand. If it wrinkles, it is probably not treated. The less a fabric wrinkles, the greater the amount of treatment. (May not apply to imported fabrics.)

Fiber Content. Before buying any fabric, check tags for fiber content. If the fabric has a strong smell, but otherwise seems acceptable, get a small sample and take it home for washing and airing. Fabrics that have been stored near polyester or fake furs (which require strong dyes) may pick up the odor of these fabrics. If the fabric still has a strong smell, do not buy it.

Corduroy Test. Try feeling it on the wrong side. With practice you can soon tell the difference between the softer, untreated fabric and the sticky, hard, treated ones. Buy half a yard to start.

REMEMBER! Test a sample from every different bolt because shipments can vary.

Glass Jar Test. Place a swatch of material in a glass jar (at least one-quart size), tighten cap and leave for thirty-six hours, and then sniff the contents. You may have an immediate reaction of nausea, nasal congestion, sneezing or coughing, a migraine headache or any change in behavior. If you are a delayed reactor and notice a problem a few hours after the test, you may have to repeat the test several times to verify that the test material is the offending substance.

Sniff Test. To be used at home when not reacting to other exposures, and preferably first thing in the morning before eating. Breathe naturally through the material for ten to fifteen minutes. If the material is deeply treated it may take only a few seconds to produce a reaction such as head pressure. Some chemical reactors, however, cannot judge treated fabric by the sniff test. If you are one who cannot judge by sniffing try to find someone who can.

Ironing Test. Ironing the material may be helpful to detect synthetics used in construction. Then try the sniff test while the material is warm.

Sleep Test. If you are still not sure, use it as a pillow overnight. Check your condition in the morning.

TIPS ON FINDING UNTREATED
NATURAL CLOTHING AND FABRICS

Special Fabrics Club. A club that will send you a swatchbook of natural, untreated fabrics, plus, periodically, sets of swatches, and information for ordering any that you may wish to try. Send $2.00 to P.O. Box 784, Skokie, Illinois 60076.

The National Cotton Council of America will provide lists of manufacturers of various products made from cotton. Write to 1030 15th Street, NW, Suite 700, Washington, D.C. 20005.

Change Your Style of Shopping. Shop at home whenever possible with catalogs and/or by telephone. If you must shop in department or specialty stores, use a folded handkerchief or a charcoal filter to prevent yourself from breathing the worst fumes. This will help you avoid reactions that cause indecision while shopping or a later "hangover." To make charcoal filter: Fold several layers of soft, untreated cotton and sew into a two-inch square leaving one edge open to form a pocket. Fill with activated charcoal and sew the ends together. Use in a handkerchief to breathe into when exposure is unavoidable.

Find a Dressmaker, Unless You Sew. Often it is easier to start from scratch and have a garment made than it is to purchase a garment which has to have the lining, inner lining, and so on, replaced.

Mainstay of Wardrobe and Furnishings. These should be natural fibers—wool, cotton, linen, silk, although some persons can tolerate viscose rayon. Even natural fibers, however, have special finishes that cause problems, and each person must check out his individual sensitivity to find compatible materials.

Import Shops. These often carry yard goods and ready-made garments of untreated cottons, silks, and woolens.

Enlist Aid of Manager. Explain that you have an allergic sensitivity to chemicals used in treatment of fabrics and to synthetic fabrics. The manager may be helpful in pointing out untreated fabrics, or in seeking a source of supply.

Read Labels Carefully. Avoid: Fiberglass (plastic is used in its construction), bonded fabrics which contain glue, materials labeled wrinkle-free, crease-resistant, Perma-press, Dura-press, stain-resistant, never-needs-ironing, Scotchgard. Note: There are a few of these which improve with the vinegar treatment, explained below.

Avoid Mothproofing. Permanent mothproofing is rarely indicated on the label. Its odor is similar to dry-cleaning fluid, with a hint of mothballs. Practically all woolens and furs in this country are mothproofed. Do not try the sniff test in store; take home on approval.

Dye Sensitivity. The dark dyes are troublesome to many persons because of chemicals used in setting the colors. Test a one-half foot of the fabric in your home before buying; wash it, and use one or more tests.

Washing Fabrics. It is imperative that your decorator or upholsterer understand that any materials chosen for drapes or slipcovers, must be *washed first*. When used for upholstering, even untreated natural fabrics should be washed to remove sizings and other chemicals used in manufacturing. This is especially true of unbleached muslin. You may need to use the vinegar treatment.

Vinegar Treatment. Use the tests for compatible fabrics (see above); however, if there is still something in the dye or manufacture of the material which is bothersome, try the following:

Use two cups of apple cider vinegar (not distilled) in a quarter tub of water (for cottons use hot water; for sheers, warm water; for washable woolens, cold water). Soak, wash thoroughly, rinse and hang out to dry. You may have to repeat this procedure one or more times. Washing with borax can be equally effective.

The vinegar treatment seldom works on Perma-press or mothproofing. It is sometimes effective, however, if the problem is something else, like Sanforizing, the dye, or the fixative used in the dye.

SOURCES

Cotton Fabrics

Ecologists Cotton Co-op, 2986 Talisman Drive, Dallas, Texas 75229. *Barrier Cloth* is available at the Co-op. Write for catalog.

Phoenix Shops (Washington, D.C., New York, Alexandria, Va.). *Handwoven Mexican Cottons*, untreated. Wide array of colors for dresses, slipcovers, draperies.

Cole's Mills, Peru, Indiana 46970. Will *quilt your fabric* on cotton batting, or quilt over other filling if requested. (Remember: down and feathers have mold, though some people can tolerate them.)

Country Curtains, Stockbridge, Mass. 01262. Coarse textured *unbleached cotton* for slacks, suits, tunics. Also white *seersucker*, bleached cotton, unbleached muslin. Catalog and swatches available. (*Some* are treated; inquire).

Carol Brown, Putney, Vermont 05346. Natural fiber fabrics, *Khadi cloth & madras* from India (expensive). Catalog available.

Wholesale firms. Write for list of 19 wholesale firms which stock *100 percent cotton merchandise.* These must be checked, however, for treatment: National Cotton Council of America, P.O. Box 12285, Memphis, Tenn. 38612.

G. Fishman & Sons, Inc., 1101-43 Des Plaines Street, Chicago, Ill. 60607. *Cotton broadcloth* 45″ wide; 100 percent linen; 100 percent China silk. Ask for samples of untreated fabrics.

West Point Pepperell, West Point, Ga. 31833. Cotton suede and cotton velour (heavy enough for coats). Ask for samples.

Homespun House, 9024 Lindblade Ave., Culver City, Calif. 90230. *Cotton* fabrics.

Linen Fabrics, Sources

Garments can be made successfully from drapery linens. Use heavier weaves for men's summer sport jackets. The best sources which are free from durable crease-resistant finishes are tablecloth linen, handkerchief linen, bedsheet linen, and pillowcase linen.

Local Department Stores. *Handkerchief* linen; *curtain* linen.

M. H. Lazarus & Co., Inc., 83 Leonard St., New York, N.Y. 10001; also Chicago. Wholesale *drapery linen;* your local store can order it.

Lee Wards, Elgin, Ill. 60120. *Ecru crewel linen* up to 70″ wide and *tablecloth* linen.

Maharam Fabric Corp., Chicago, Ill. Wholesale *drapery* linen. Your local store can order it.

E. H. & A. C. Friedrich's Co., 10 Sullivan Street, New York, New York 10012. *Untreated linen* with vegetable sizing; write for samples.

G. Fishman & Sons, Inc., 1101-43 Des Plaines Street, Chicago, Ill. 60607. *Untreated linen;* samples.

Silk Fabrics

Silk is a good basic fabric because problems encountered can be removed and/or counteracted. If untreated, silk usually water-spots. Remove the formaldehyde used in the processing of most silk by several washings in hot, soapy water. (Any loss of body can be replaced to some extent by using gum arabic starch).

Fabric Centre, 107 Downie Street, Stratford, Ontario, Canada. *Silk & velvet* swatches available.

Local department stores. *China* silk and *raw* silk.

Ibec Thailand Limited, Maneeya Bldg., 51812 Ploenchet Road, Bangkok, Thailand, Post Box 936. *Thai silks*—beautiful prints in light and heavy weights. Very reliable firm, and less expensive than local sources.

G. Dean Morgan, 4276 Los Palos, Palo Alto, Calif. 94306. Five weights of *Thai silk.*

Thai Silk, 393 Main Street, Los Altos, California 94022. Silks (and cottons) from Thailand, the Orient, and the Philippines.

Carol Brown, Putney, Vermont 05346: Tussah *raw silk, Siamese silk.*

Ying Tai Fashions, 88A Nathan Road, 1st Floor, Kowloon, P.O. Box K-2251, Hong Kong. Silk *piece goods;* catalog available; very reliable.

G. Fishman & Sons, Inc., 1101-43 Des Plaines Street, Chicago, Illinois 60607. *China silk, Shantung silk;* ask for samples.

Froerman Yard Goods, 215 W. Jackson Blvd., Chicago, Illinois 60606: *Silks;* ask for samples.

Viscose Rayon

Derived from wood pulp or cotton linters as raw material, viscose rayon is tolerated by some persons who cannot tolerate other rayon fabrics which are produced synthetically. Viscose has a rough feel to it, and fabric finishes may be washed off, whereas acetate, for instance, is slippery and the finish can never be removed because it is put on through a carbon-bonding finish.

Brand names are: Avril, Bemberg, Coloray, Colorspun, Supioni, Enka Rayon, Fortisan, Spunlo, Zantrel.

Woolen Fabrics

Most woolen fabric manufactured in the United States is moth-proofed. Occasionally a manufacturer, if requested, will produce a bolt of fabric that has not been mothproofed. Many of these sources for untreated fabrics are foreign.

Anousso E. Madoupa, Mykonos, Greece. *Dress lengths* of handwoven silk and wool; ask for samples.

Avoca Handweavers Ltd., Avoca Co., Wicklew, Ireland. *Handwoven yard goods* in solids, heathers, checks, light coating weights. State color preference when ordering samples.

Clansman Tweed Co., Ltd., 9 Kenneth Street, Stornoway, Isle of Lewis, Scotland: *Harris tweeds* (which usually are sprayed if requested by retail establishments; specify untreated). Also, blankets, stoles, knee rugs.

Gaeltarra Eireann, 34 Westland Row, Dublin, Ireland. *Coating fabric* in classic twill and lightweight wools. Beautiful tweeds 56″ wide; reasonable.

Paisleys Ltd., Jamaica Street, Glasgow, Scotland. Over *400 woolen tartans,* specify untreated; samples and catalog.

Carol Brown, Putney, Vermont 05346: *Tweeds.* Prices sent upon request.

Leiter's Fabrics, 4448 Belleview Street, Kansas City, Mo. 64111. *Designer Fabrics,* specify untreated; wide widths.

Briggs & Littles Woolen Mill, York Mills, Harvey Station, N.B., Canada. Specify untreated; ask for samples.

Knit & Purl, Randhurst Center, Mount Prospect, Illinois. *Knitting yarn,* color-coordinated to *tweed, check* or *solid* yard goods which they arrange to have made into skirts.

Springfield Woolen Mills, Springfield, Minn. 56087. Get brochure on reworking your old *comforters* with new wool, or making wool batting from old woolen materials.

Moffat Hand Loom Weavers, Ladyknowe, Moffat, Dumfrieshere, Scotland: Tartans, tweeds, plaids, color-coordinated with sweaters, yarns.

Wool Knitting Yarns

Knitting as a hobby provides warm, untreated, undyed, unmothproofed hats, mittens, socks, sweaters, even blankets.

Silver Shuttle, 1301 35th Street, NW, Washington, D.C. Undyed, unmothproofed alpaca yarn in natural shades of soft white, tans, grays, and browns. Write for information.

Knit & Purl, Randhurst Center, Mount Prospect, Illinois. *Rygja* natural knitting yarn with sheep oils in it. Austrian medium weight yarn; knitting yarn color-coordinated to tweed, check or solid yard goods.

Alaska Native Arts & Crafts Co-op, Ass'n, Inc., Juneau, Alaska. *Bone crochet hooks.* Seal, $4.00; Bear, $4.00; catalog of crafts.

Moffat Hand Loom Weavers, Ladyknowe, Moffat, Dumfrieshere, Scotland. *Untreated knitting yarns;* send for brochure.

The Golf Links, St. Andrews, Scotland. *Yarns;* specify untreated.

Wm. Condon & Sons, POB 129, Charlottetown, Prince Edward Island, Canada. *Natural yarns* (light oil treatment washes away).

Mrs. Christine Macleod, Hillside Cottage, Ardhasaig, Isle of Harris, Outer Hebrides, Scotland. *Harris Knitting Wools,* Harris tweeds, some with natural oils; ask for samples.

Handcraft House, 1942 Marine Drive, North Vancouver, B.C., Canada. *Wool chart,* 50¢; catalog, 50¢.

Tahki Imports, 336 West End Avenue, New York, N.Y. 10023. *Sheep's wool* from Greece, five natural shades.

The Mannings, Creative Crafts, East Berlin, Pa. 17316. *Yarns;* catalog available.

Folklorico, P.O. Box 625, Palo Alto, Calif. 94302. *Mexican wool, Australian angora*, natural colors.

Macramé & Weaving Supply Co., 63 East Adams Street, Chicago, Illinois 60603. *Avanti Primitive, Loop mohair*.

Old Mill Yarn, P.O. Box 115, Eaton Rapids, Michigan 48827. Untreated *wool yarns*.

Contessa Yarns, P.O. Box 37, Lebanon, Conn. 06249. Untreated *wool yarns*.

Dyes

Whenever possible use natural dyes. Dyes may be a problem and there are no available tests. Many foreign fabrics, such as Thai silks and Indian cottons, which were once safe are now suspect because of the newer dyes used. Also, turpentine is sometimes used as a pesticide when Indian cottons are shipped, because it is cheaper than DDT. The turpentine is virtually impossible to remove. If DDT is present, it is usually in the form of a gray powder.

Home Dyes. Sassafras tea can be used to dye white fabrics a pinkish shrimp color. Put a small amount of tea into a pot with water in it, bring it to a boil, and dip fabric into it. Be careful not to let the fabric fold while wet, or it will be unevenly colored. Leave submerged or dip until dark enough. Lay fabric out flat to dry. The dye does not fade after it is washed.

Try experimenting with the scouting method of dyeing (beets, onion skins, black walnuts, butternuts), methods of dyeing used by the pioneers.

Screen Process Supplies Mfg. Co., 1199 E. 12th Street, Oakland, California 94606. *Vat* dyes for cotton or linen, type 4; clear extender.

Mrs. G. C. McDonald, 620 Sierra Drive, S.E., Albuquerque, New Mex. 87108. *Hopi* Dyes.

For vegetable dyes, write to: Earth Guild, 149 Putnam Avenue, Cambridge, Mass. 02134.

For information about dyes, order "Natural Plant Dye," Handbook #72 which includes instructions for the beginning dyer, a bibliography of books on dyeing, and a list of dye plant suppliers. Send check for $1.50 to Brooklyn Botanic Garden, 1000 Washington Avenue, Brooklyn, New York 11225.

TIPS FOR THE DO-IT-YOURSELFER OR PROFESSIONAL SEAMSTRESS

If you choose to work with a dressmaker, a professional seamstress, or a tailor on your new nontoxic wardrobe, it might be wise to have your professional helper read this section of the book before beginning.

Sewing or having your clothes made widens your choice of clothing. Sewing with nontoxic materials requires special procedures that even an experienced dressmaker would not necessarily be expected to know.

All clothing, whether off-the-rack or designed especially for you, must meet the following criteria:

1. Select 100 percent pure cotton, silk, or linen. Some wools also may be tolerated.

2. When possible, the dyes should be natural.

3. The fabric must be free of chemical treatments: mothproofing, bonding to a lining (glue is used to attach the fabrics), Scotchgarding, or any other process that prevents staining, and any wrinkle-preventing treatments such as Perma-press or Dura-press.

4. All notions, linings, and interfacings must be chemical-free.

Always wash the fabric before cutting to get out any residue from other fabrics and to shrink the fabric *before* it becomes a garment.

All fabrics for allergic people should be stored separately in cardboard boxes—never placed in plastic, and never near polyester or other synthetic fabrics.

Sewing with Cotton. Cotton is a versatile fabric that comes in many weights and weaves from lightweight batiste, lawn, and organdy to muslin, percale, piqué, corduroy, denim, terry cloth, and mattress ticking. It is easy to sew, dyes well, and its dyes are less likely to be toxic than those used on linen or wool. Cotton wrinkles easily, however, and is likely to be treated for this. If the fabric is not marked, you can easily check for treatment. If cotton wrinkles under even slight pressure, it has not been treated.

Pesticides used in growing cotton often remain in the fabric. Try soaking, then wash it in vinegar or borax.

Barrier Cloth. We know that toxic mothers usually give birth to toxic babies. Mothers who smoke and are exposed in other ways to harmful chemicals during their pregnancy run an enormous risk of making the unborn infant susceptible to allergies resulting in colic, rashes, nasal stuffiness and many other infant complaints which could be avoided. Be kind to your baby. Don't create more problems for him. Avoid using plastic pants and disposable diapers. Instead use pure cotton diapers, washed in borax, rinsed in apple vinegar, and protected by wet-proof pants made of barrier cloth. Just cut the barrier cloth to size, sew elastic bands around the waist and the legs and you have wet-proof pants. For baby's bed make a mattress cover of barrier cloth and cotton quilting.

Sewing with Silk. Many dressmakers have never sewn with silk, which requires special handling procedures. Sewing with silk is frustrating, if not impossible, if these procedures are not followed, but with care and a little practice anyone can do it without too much trouble.

1. Use a pair of very sharp, straight scissors. Even the sharpest pinking shears will not cut silk properly. Test the scissors blades by running them along a pair of old stockings.

2. Use only sharp, silk-dressmaking pins. Test needles on a scrap of silk. Generally, the thinner the needle, the better. If you are unsure about the size of the sewing machine needles, ask your fabric store or sewing machine sales representative. Select a needle that will not pull on the fabric and that will not leave a hole.

3. Adjust the top and bottom tensions, testing with a piece of silk. Again, if you have trouble, visit your sewing machine sales representative. You will have to adjust the throat plate for silk. This is the plate on which the fabric is pulled as it is being sewn. The teeth on the plate can be adjusted for a perfect grip of the fabric.

4. If the material still slips, sew through tissue or other lightweight paper. The paper is easy to remove later.

5. Zig-zag all seams and edges to prevent raveling.

6. Silk thread must be used.

China silk makes beautiful lingerie and blouses, but it is next to impossible to iron. Avoid designs with fancy cuffs or sleeves. Bias-cut bows and ties may be used if they are detachable when the rest of the garment is laundered. Buy an additional quarter to half yard of fabric and make up several bows. *Do not* make up the bows without washing first; China silk changes texture just slightly when washed, and so the bow will look foreign to the blouse if the fabric is not washed at least once prior to cutting and sewing.

Linen and Wool. Linen and wool can sometimes be tolerated, but there are no fabric tests for them. Try these fabrics in small quantities. American wool is usually mothproofed.

Notions. Linings, interfacings and notions must be chemical free. Here are some important pointers:

1. **Linings and interfacings** must be of cotton, silk or wool, which eliminates most products sold for this purpose. Where warmth is desired, try a cotton thermal blanket, stay-stitched and cross-stitched to lightweight flannel. Viyella (50 percent cotton/50 percent wool) used for men's shirts, when available, makes a warm lining.

2. **Buttons** may be metal, pure mother-of-pearl, wood (unfinished), or porcelain (unpainted).

3. **Zippers** must be made of metal. These are often available in bulk form from larger sewing shops.

4. **Elastic** generally cannot be tolerated; however, many very sensitive patients can use elastic if it is enclosed in a casing. If elastic cannot be tolerated at all, try cotton elastic. Unfortunately, this elastic has very little stretch, and a creative seamstress may find it better to design a garment without elastic by using extra buttons, snaps, or zippers. Drawstrings of an acceptable fabric give many garments the flexibility of elastic.

5. **Thread** should be pure cotton or silk. However, many extremely sensitive persons can tolerate polyester thread used on cotton knit garments. (Cotton thread breaks under stress; polyester has some stretch). If you cannot tolerate polyester thread at all, use zig-zag or chain stitches on any parts of the knit garment that can be stretched.

6. **Belt backings** are generally not tolerable. Try folding several layers of unbleached muslin to the desired width. Stay-stitch to hold the layers, then use as a backing. (Muslin will not be as stiff as belt backing.)

If a very wide or stiff belt is preferred, cut a piece of wire screen about three-quarters of an inch narrower and shorter than the muslin backing. Sandwich the screen inside the muslin, carefully placing it so you can sew around the muslin without sewing through the wire. Hammer large nails through the muslin and wire where the belt eyelets will be placed. Enlarge the holes so they can easily accommodate the eyelet punch.

TIPS ON READY-MADE CLOTHING

Vinegar Rinse. Often a vinegar rinse or a washing with borax (if you find the vinegar smell hard to rinse out) will remove the odor from chemicals used in manufacturing or storing. This rinse also will sometimes remove light Perma-press treatments.

Cultivate the Thrift Shop Habit. Stores such as the Salvation Army and Goodwill sometimes yield rare discoveries, particularly because the extra care required for silks, untreated woolens, and all cotton garments make these fabrics less desirable to those more interested in convenience than health.

Resell Your Mistakes. You will make mistakes and from time to time buy a garment that cannot be worn. Sell it through the thrift shop or a garage sale. Or store the garment for a year—the toxicity may eventually disappear.

Clothing Sources Change. Even before this book is published, some of the items recommended, which have been reliable for years, may have changed and now contain synthetics or have undesirable finishes. For that reason everything must be tested for you—and you alone. Let the merchant know your disappointment in synthetics and your need for natural fabrics; he may be helpful in finding you compatible clothing.

Sources of Material. You can greatly expand your fabric choices if you shop in foreign speciality shops and drapery stores. Elegant coats for under $15 have been made from cotton bedspreads from India. Look in linen departments for tablecloths that may be turned into blouses, beach coverups or dresses, or look for bright linens or terrycloth towels that can be converted to skirts or playwear.

Do you have the thrift shop habit? You might find quilts that can be turned into hostess skirts or robes; an old full dress of pure silk that has enough yardage to turn it into a new dress. You may even find a fur coat that is coming back in style, and is not treated as are new coats. If the fur is in good condition, an old coat can be made to look like new.

In addition, search the want ads under clothing or garage sales. In most cities there are also several publications that are nothing *but* want ads.

Furs and Leathers. Most furs in the United States are mothproofed. Some imported furs are also mothproofed if American buyers request it. Also, a chemical treatment is used on fur that makes it undesirable for many persons. The Australian lamb coat, however, is tolerated well by chemically sensitive persons. Order from: Cornelius Furs, Box 3960 G.P.O., Sydney, Australia, 2001.

American suede has tar in it, which explains why many allergic persons cannot tolerate it. There is a tailor in Istanbul who will make suede suits, skirts, jackets lined in silk or cotton. Ask for the finest quality suede—not mothproofed; send body measurements and $20 deposit; Vezir Han Cad, Lutfu Han No. 60, Cemberlitas, Istanbul.

Women's Clothing

Hosiery. Agilon all-nylon panty hose (available at Lord & Taylor's and other department stores) can be tolerated by some patients. Pure silk panty hose (expensive) now available at Lord & Taylor's.

Solaris brand, white, 100 percent pure silk undersocks are available in ski shops. Wear them under pure cotton socks (to keep your feet warm).

Ultrason by Berkshire is well tolerated by many sensitive patients.

Lismore Hosiery Company, 334 Grand Street, New York City, 10002. Cotton knee socks, rayon, cotton, or lisle stockings.

Bergdorf Goodman, 754 Fifth Avenue, New York, New York 10019. Pure silk stockings.

Try these cotton clothing items: Buster Brown socks, cotton nightgowns and slips, 100 percent cotton chenille robes, Belle Sharmeer nylon panty hose with panty lined in cotton, Chansonette Maidenform bras, French T-shirts.

Underwear. Catalog stores (Sears, Montgomery Ward). Cotton garter belts, terry-cloth bathrobes, cotton panties, cotton flannel nightgowns (avoid deep dyes), cotton slips.

Maidenform has a bra made of cotton knit. Bali is another brand name of a cotton bra.

Your dressmaker can make you slips, bras, pajamas from silk or viscose rayon. Custom-made bras—yellow pages, local telephone directory.

Dresses, Blouses, Slack-suits. Robert Reis Brand, cotton, ribbed turtleneck sweaters (men's furnishings departments).

Andean Products, Box 472, Cuenca, Ecuador. Hand-embroidered, natural cotton dresses, blouses, men's shirts and accessories; catalog available (avoid macramé purse).

May Fashion House, Deck 1, 146 Ocean Terminal, Kowloon, Hong Kong. Silk dresses, woolen suits (knits), pant suits (reasonable); ask for catalog.

The Phoenix, 301 Cameron, Alexandria, Virginia 22314. (Also, N.Y. City, Washington, D.C. store.) Natural Mexican cotton dresses, blouses, accessories, beautiful hand embroidery.

Tom's Gift Shoppe, 665 Queen Street, Niagara Falls, Canada. Silk and cotton blouses.

Skyr, Anba, Profile brands of 100 percent cotton, long-sleeved shirts at ski-wear shops.

Mission Village, Box 211, Freeport, New York 11520. Black and white handwoven cotton jackets from Guatemala; handwoven cotton dress and skirt lengths, beautiful colors.

Kori, 13 Mitropoleos Street, Athens, Greece. Producers and designers of handwoven dresses.

Windfall, Main Street, Sharon Springs, N.Y. 13459. Beautiful cotton dresses, short and long; catalog available.

J. Jill, Ltd., Great Barrington, Mass. 01230. Cotton dresses and blouses, robes, very attractive; catalog available.

The Talbots, 164 North Street, Hingham, Mass. 02043. Cotton velveteen blazer (ask about lining), cotton robes, nightgowns, skirts, shearling-lined slippers (beware of dyed *leather*).

Coats, Jackets, Sweaters. Moffat Hand Loom Weavers, Ladyknowe, Moffat, Dumfrieshere, Scotland. Untreated woolen dresses, ensembles, skirts, sweaters.

Antartex Sheepskins, Loch Lomond, Scotland. Sheepskin coats, jackets, mitts, slippers, hats; catalog available, 139 East 76th Street, New York, N.Y.

Irish Cottage Industries, 18 Dawson Street, Dublin, Ireland. Fairisle multicolored yoke sweaters, natural wool, handknit; Aran natural wool sweaters in off-white or colors; ask for "oiled wool" to get untreated sweater.

Cowichan Trading Company, 589 Johnson Street, Victoria, British Columbia, Canada. Natural, raw sheep's wool, handknit into beautiful Indian designs. Also, toques, tams, socks, mittens.

R. S. Duncan & Co., 30 Chapel Street, Bradford 1, England. Untreated *washable* woolen cardigans, raglan-sleeve, pullover sweaters; matching skirts or material to make skirts. The ready-made skirts appear to have a synthetic lining. Sweaters are *very* inexpensive.

Carol Brown, Putney, Vermont 05346. Handknit sweaters.

Riding apparel stores. Corduroy jodphurs, heavy weight, usually untreated.

Catalog stores. Cotton knit slacks, all colors; Lee's corduroy jeans.

Icemart, Keflavik International Airport, Iceland. Handknit sweaters of natural-color wool, skirts, slacks.

Natural, undyed, and untreated sweaters, socks, and mittens may be obtained from the Cowichan Trading Company, 589 Johnson Street, Victoria, British Columbia, Canada. Phone: 383-0321. The natural oils are retained, thus giving the garments a waterproof quality.

Shoes. Sources of women's shoes without synthetic innersoles or synthetic linings are rare. If the shoe has synthetic materials, it will have stamped on the sole the words "man-made materials." Linings can sometimes be removed, using a very sharp artist's knife. The innersoles can be replaced with leather innersoles.

Dr. Scholl's sandals. Only some are "all" leather.

Bloom's Shoe Shop, 311 6th Avenue, New York, N.Y. 10014. Vegetable tanned Buff-Alohe sandals (also children's); catalog available.

Brockton Shoe Company, Brockton, Mass. Manufacturer of women's all-leather golf shoes.

L. L. Bean, Inc., Freeport, Maine 04032. 8″ high leather boots lined in sheepskin.

Department stores. California Cobblers, all leather; Bandolino, leather lining (women can also wear men's leather slipper lined in sheepskin); Amalfi all-leather, Italian-made shoes.

Quoddy Moccasins, 443 Western Avenue, South Portland, Maine 04106. Leather moccasins, sandals, shearling-lined slippers, boots.

Antartex, 139 East 76th Street, New York, N.Y. Leather boots lined with sheepskin (British sizes).

Men's Clothing

Shirts. Eddie Bauer, P.O. Box 3700, Seattle, Washington 98124. Warm chamois cotton; colors; catalog available.

Ascot Chang Company, 34 Kimberly Road, Kowloon, Hong Kong. Many untreated fabrics, tailored to order; catalog available.

Supermarkets and drug stores. Cotton sweat shirts; white, colors.

A. Garstand & Company, Ltd., 213 Preston New Road, Blackburn, England. Cotton, silk, fine wool; catalog available.

L. L. Bean, Inc., Freeport, Maine 04032. Wool, Viyella (cotton and wool), cotton. Catalog.

J. Packard, Ltd., Terre Haute, Indiana 47808. 100 percent cotton made-to-order. Request substitution of cotton interlining for synthetic in the collars.

Trousers, Walking Shorts. Burton's Clothing Store, Dundee, Scotland. Wool slacks, beautifully tailored. Write for information.

L. L. Bean, Inc., Freeport, Maine 04032. Wool slacks; catalog available.

Department stores. Ask for Levi's, Canvas Spikes, blue jeans, McGregor tennis shorts.

Suits. Brooks Bros., Washington, D.C.; New York; Chicago. Cotton seersucker (imported from England), tailor-made untreated wool (Brook-Ease brand); catalog available.

Other men's clothing stores. Look for cotton/wool suits; cotton/silk and silk/wool.

Coats, Jackets, Sweaters, Sleepwear, Underwear. L. L. Bean, Inc., Freeport, Maine 04032. Corduroy English walking jacket, slacks.

Department and catalog stores. Cotton sleep shirts, jockey underwear, cotton leisure suits.

Sun Valley Mail Order, Sun Valley, Idaho 83353. Fisherman knit cotton shirts, wool slacks, caps. Toll free mail order 1-800-635-5313. (Women's clothing, too.)

Icemart Mail Order House, Keflavik International Airport, Iceland. Untreated wool sweaters in natural colors; blankets are mothproofed.

Holubar, Box 7, Boulder, Colorado 80302. Cotton-knit turtleneck shirts, long cotton underwear; catalog available.

Eddie Bauer, P.O. Box 3700, Seattle, Washington 98124. Long underwear of Viyella. Pendleton hosiery, 100 percent wool, dark colors, machine washable; catalog available.

Irish Cottage Industries, 18 Dawson Street, Dublin, Ireland. Aran natural wool sweaters in off-white or colors; ask for "oiled wool" to get untreated sweaters.

R. S. Duncan & Company, 30 Chapel Street, Bradford 1, England. Untreated, washable woolen sweaters. Very nice, inexpensive!

Daniel Low & Company, 231 Essex Street, Salem, Mass. 01970. Cotton corduroy slacks, polo shirts, bathrobes of cotton flannel.

Norm Thompson, 1805 N.W. Thurman, Portland, Oregon 97209. Coats, sweaters, slacks; catalog available.

Shoes

Daniel Low & Company. Suede leather moccasin with arch support, made in Spain.

Quoddy Moccasins, 443 Western Avenue, South Portland, Maine 04106. Leather moccasins, slippers; catalog available.

Brockton Shoe Company, Brockton, Massachusetts. Leather shoes, vegetable tanned; catalog available.

Bloom's Shoe Shop, 311 6th Avenue, New York, N.Y. 10014. Buff Alohe, vegetable tanned; catalog available.

Eddie Bauer, P.O. Box 3700, Seattle, Washington 98124. Scotch grain chukka boots; catalog available.

CHAPTER 27

Home Furnishings

ANNE, a woman who previously had lived in her house without difficulty suddenly began to feel ill. Every room in the house seemed to cause her trouble. This condition had begun shortly after she had taken her summer home furniture out of storage and moved it into her year-round home.

The summer home furniture had never caused a problem before, though, so that couldn't be the source.

After a certain amount of sleuthing, the mystery was solved. A clinical ecologist discovered that the storage company had followed its standard procedure of spraying furniture with insecticide before moving and storing it. The furniture was indeed the "guilty party."

As a result, all the furniture which had been carefully made to order for her suddenly became useless. Anne was forced to get rid of it.

We know of others who have made such costly mistakes. One of them, Ellen, now tells salesmen, "Don't do me any favors. Don't try to save me any money." In retrospect, she can laugh at some of the incidents that caused her so many problems. At the time that they happened, however, they were disturbing to her. Even now, she says, she laughs with a lump in her throat and a tear in her eye.

Ellen is one of those persons who "never had any allergies." She was just slightly bothered by deodorants. When she was furnishing a new apartment, her sister mentioned to her that since she had this mild sensitivity, perhaps she should buy an acrylic carpet rather than the wool one that she was selecting. And besides, "It will cost you less money," she said.

Ellen, always reasonable, decided on the acrylic. Nine months later, when she was diagnosed as severely sensitive, she discovered she was highly allergic to acrylic materials and other synthetics, but not to wool.

Her next purchase for her apartment was her draperies. She chose beautiful antique silk shantung. The interior decorator said, "Since you're spending so much money, why not add another $100 and have them lined with a special material that will guard them from sun damage?"

The silk was fine. The chemically treated lining was not. Ellen was highly sensitive to it.

Her custom-made sleep sofa was designed to meet her specific needs. The designer said to her, "You are putting so much money into this couch, for $35 more you can have it treated to resist stains."

There was nothing in that sofa that made her ill except the well-advertised product used to make the material stain-resistant. Now, ten years later, she still cannot sit on that sofa when she visits the relative to whom she gave it.

Thus her motto, "Don't do me any favors. Don't try to save me any money."

Even the less costly mistakes which need only minor adjustments can cause as much discomfort. For example, Jack W. hated to start each day—he felt miserable.[1] "In the mornings," he said, "I felt as if I didn't even want to get up. I had a postnasal drip but the major problem was that I felt so disagreeable I was not fit to be around anyone until about 10:30 in the morning." After a consultation with a clinical ecologist, he got rid of his polyester mattress and immediately his problems disappeared. His good disposition also returned.

Cotton mattress pads are hard to find, but a felted cotton pad exists which looks much like a blanket and does not produce the problem that polyester causes. If a cotton blanket or pad cannot be located, an additional cotton fitted sheet or two might be used instead of a pad.

One knowledgeable man thought he had made his bedroom free of polyester, yet he seemed to be having trouble. He checked his bed, sure that his sheets and pillow cases were all cotton, and found to his surprise that they were 50 percent polyester. Amazingly, within a few days after the bedding was replaced, a long-standing dandruff problem almost disappeared.

"For several years," he said, "I had been plagued with heavy white dandruff-like fur over the bald part of my head. In the mornings I would sometimes wash my head carefully or rub it off with a cloth until it was clean. In half an hour or so the white fur would be back.

"After changing to cotton sheets, the problem just disappeared and did not return."

Beware of polyester and other synthetics in batting used in pillows, mattress pads and upholstery. Allergic people mistakenly substitute synthetic pillows for feather pillows not knowing that the synthetics could be worse for them.

Upholstery

The allergic patient often cannot tolerate polyurethane foam, treated fabrics, synthetic fabrics, plastic upholstery, foam rubber. Each item needs to be tested personally.

Upholstery Materials. Remove foam or polyurethane, plastic and treated coverings from furniture; replace with innerspring and cotton padding. (Be sure to use plain, white quilting cotton; the "natural" cotton for upholstery is treated.) Furniture may be upholstered in white cotton over which one could use slipcovers of linen, Mexican cotton, unbleached muslin with cotton braid trim, corduroy, cotton velveteen (if not flameproofed). Wash *all* material first. Do not replace canvas strips unless absolutely necessary; wash new strips many times to remove kerosene. (See vinegar treatment, page 234.)

Arrange with your decorator to let you wash all upholstery materials and provide white cotton. Your materials must be isolated in his shop, and placed as far as possible from treated and synthetic materials. Otherwise, they will absorb chemicals like a sponge and will have to be aired for months. An understanding decorator will arrange to do your furniture for you in a minimum length of time in order to get it in and out of the shop as quickly as possible.

Materials may be purchased from:

Greet Fabrics, 150 Midland Avenue, Port Chester, N.Y. or Merchandise Mart, Chicago, 82 percent linen and 18 percent rayon.

Myron Paul Originals, Merchandise Mart, Chicago, pure upholstery linen, also tweeds.

Berea College, Log House Sales, Box 778, Campus, Berea, Kentucky 40403. Write for samples and prices.

Curtains

100 percent cotton lace curtains can be obtained from HB, 597 Farmington Avenue, Hartford, Conn. 06105. Swatches, 25 cents; catalog, 75 cents.

Bleached white ruffled muslin curtains pre-shrunk: tiebacks from 45" to 72" long, or from 81" to 90" long; tiers from 20" to 40" long; Matching valance from 11" to 74".

Order from Country Curtains, Red Lion Inn, Dept. 74, Stockbridge, Massachusetts 01262.

Draperies

(See linen and cotton fabric sources, Chapter 25.) Wash all fabrics before they are made into draperies. If the decorator washes the fabrics for you, make sure that he uses your soap.

Fabrics may be purchased from:

Flexalum, Central Smithway Co., 2829 N. Natoma Ave., Chicago, Ill. 60634. Woven aluminum draperies and shades.

M. H. Lazarus & Co., Inc., 83 Leonard St., New York, N.Y. 10013 (Chicago, also). Wholesale drapery linen which can be ordered by your local store.

E. H. & A. C. Friedrich's Co., 10 Sullivan St., New York, N.Y. 10012. Untreated linen with vegetable sizing.

The Phoenix, Washington, D.C., Alexandria, Va., New York City. Natural Mexican cottons, colors, patterns.

Variety Stores. Unbleached and bleached muslin, ideal for curtains, sheets, slips.

Lamps

Look for 100 percent silk shades (washable). Metal, glass, or silk shades are recommended since heated plastic is troublesome for the allergic person. Avoid fluorescent lamps, which produce ozone. Glass shields help.

Furniture

Tables and Benches. Rattan, wood of all kinds, glass, aluminum, and Formica, mounted on metal legs. (Be sure to cover underside of table and benches with Formica, also, to prevent glue from volatizing through the bottom.)

Chairs and Sofas. Reupholster present furniture. Purchase colonial, Scandinavian or modern styles with loose cushions. If cushions are filled with foam rubber or synthetics, have new cushions made by an upholsterer, using springs and white cotton batting.

Yugoslavian corded chairs, rockers, and love seats are available from import stores. Also available are several kinds of fiber and rattan. Interesting furniture with sheepskin seat and back, reasonably priced, is available from Carlson & Reicke, Sceacagen 33, Stockholm, Sweden. (Check that it is free from mothproofing.)

Garage Sales. Do not overlook neighborhood garage sales, where it is possible to pick up older furniture without fresh chemical treatments or synthetics. When buying any second-hand products, make sure they have not been sprayed with insecticides.

Accessories. Items such as these cut down the plastic exposure in your home: woven waste baskets, laundry baskets, hemp place mats. Useful, untreated household accessories may be found at stores specializing in import goods.

Rugs. Avoid carpeting. The mats under carpeting are highly toxic, most woolen carpeting is mothproofed, and untreated cotton looks shabby and will not hold up well. Even if you can find attractive carpeting, it is not advisable, for dust and mold cannot be cleaned from the carpet. For rugs, use untreated cotton and unmothproofed wools. Some sources to explore are:

Dellinger, Rome, Georgia 30161. Manufacturers of custom cotton carpet on special order.

Flokati-Hellas, care of Mr. Kostas Staikopoulos, Athens, Greece. This manufacturer/exporter can furnish white, long-haired, natural wool rugs that have not been treated. Specify that they be sent airmail, to avoid absorbing chemicals on ship.

Navajo Arts & Crafts Guild, Window Rock, Arkansas. 100 percent wool rugs; fast vegetable dyes.

Edward Lacey Mills, Inc., Fairmont, Georgia. Reversible cotton rug for bath or bedroom.

Indian Trading Post, Wisconsin Dells, Wisconsin. Navajo rugs preserved with onion skins.

Apelian Rug Company, 2900 Central, Evanston, Illinois. Cotton carpeting made in Tennessee.

Harmony Carpet Corporation, 979 Third Avenue, New York, N.Y. 10022. Natural Berber rug designs in wool, representing Spanish, French, Scotch, and African primitive designs (through your decorator).

Bedroom Furnishings

Mattresses. Should be free from chemical finishes without sizing and chemical odor retardants or layers of foam or polyurethane. The legislation requiring flameproofing of mattresses can now be waived with a doctor's statement. If it is necessary to quote the regulation that permits this waiver, it can be found as para. 1632 "Standard for Flammability of mattresses (and mattress pads) (FS 4-72 of the Consumer Product Safety Commission, Flammable Fabrics Act Regulation.)" The amendment is para. 1632. 1.

With the proper statement, a mattress can be ordered to your specifications from Hotel Mattress Suppliers and from the Artel Bedding Co., 1573 Ellinwood St., Des Plaines, Illinois.

Until such time as the government allows anyone, even without a physician's statement, to buy a toxic-free mattress, it is suggested that you buy a mattress cover made of barrier cloth (see page 230).

Pillows. Fill a pillow cover (cotton) with soft baby diapers, turkish towels, or towels torn in strips. A soft cotton receiving blanket or white cotton batting can be used. Freshen weekly in electric dryer. Some persons who cannot tolerate feathers *can* tolerate goose down pillows.

Blankets. Try Goodwill or the Salvation Army for old blankets. These can be washed, and enclosed in a cotton blanket cover for a warm quilt. Avoid electric blankets—the plastic wires are troublesome when heated.

From time to time cotton thermoweave blankets are available from catalog companies. You can sometimes find them in department stores. Most of them have a nylon border which can be removed. If the blanket is unfinished, you may wish to attach a cotton border to replace the one you have removed.

Coles Mills, Peru, Indiana. Will quilt your fabric on cotton batting or your own filling if you request it.

Berea College, Berea, Kentucky. Infants' woolen blankets, couch throws; catalog available.

Clansman Tweed Company, Ltd., 9 Kenneth Street, Stornoway, Isle of Lewis, Scotland. Woolen blankets untreated, if requested. (Usually treated when ordered through stores in the United States.)

Moffat Hand Loom Weavers, Ladyknowe, Moffat, Dumfrieshere, Scotland. Mohair blankets and rugs (specify untreated).

Springfield Woolen Mills. Springfield, Minnesota 56087. Brochure available on reworking your old comforters with new wool, or making wool batting from old woolen materials.

Sheets and Mattress Pads. The availability of 100 percent cotton bedding varies from year to year. Wamsutta makes a 100 percent cotton sheet, but it is expensive. Garage sales turn up many good 100 percent cotton sheets. If you have difficulty finding bedding, speak to the buyers in your department store. If they can't help, it is available at the Ecologist's Cotton Co-op (see page 234).

For information write: The National Cotton Council of America, P.O. Box 12285, Memphis, Tennessee; or write Memphis Cotton Wives, P.O. Box 22067, Memphis, Tennessee 38122 for shopping guide for 100 percent cotton items.

Bedspreads of 100 percent cotton are easy to find. Avoid the label, Perma-press, and Indian dyes, which seem to hold a kerosene treatment that will not wash out.

Make your own bedspreads from cottons, if desired, using the *white* cotton quilt batting (prewashed, or pure wool batting).

Accessories

Waste Baskets. Natural woven material or metal.

Clocks and Clock Radios. Remember that heated plastic causes trouble. Use travel alarm, or transistor clock. Keep clock-radio at a distance from your sleeping area. Avoid having a lighted clock in your bedroom. While the fumes they give off are usually not detectable, they have been found to make many people ill.

Books, Magazines, Newspapers. Keep sleeping area as free as possible from plastic book covers and kerosene-soaked printed pages. Let someone else read papers and books first, or air outside. When you retire, remove reading material as far as possible from the air you breathe at night.

Closets and Dresser Drawers. Control fumes by using filters made from activated charcoal covered with cotton. Air woolens at least once a week to avoid moths. Wash cottons often. Air enclosed spaces generously.

CHAPTER 28

Cosmetics and Toiletries

WHILE MANY products are referred to as hypoallergenic, so many patients have reported illness from them that doctors have suggested these individuals may have been reacting to one or more ingredients in the cosmetics. It may have been coloring and dye or preservatives or coal-tar petroleum products or alcohol or witch hazel, to name the most likely suspects.

The cosmetic recipes and suggestions given here represent formulas devised by patients and/or doctors and shared with us. We selected those most frequently reported as helpful. Again, no product is safe for everyone.

Prevention. It is not always possible to tell which toxins are present in various cosmetics because of the necessary secrecy of the formulas. Therefore, for preventive purposes, it is recommended that you prepare your own makeup whenever possible.

Many allergic patients find that while they must use organic products internally, they can sometimes externally apply mixtures containing nonorganic products. However, they cannot tolerate external application of a food to which they have an allergic reaction.

The only products mentioned in this chapter are those that have been used without difficulty by many extremely sensitive people. As with everything else in this book, the allergic patient is cautioned to test them carefully, preferably under the supervision of a doctor.

Application. For face and neck care, wash your face before you apply any mask or astringent. So many people have such sensitive skins that upon first use, anything applied should be washed off after two minutes to determine whether the ingredients can be tolerated. For this reason, too, there are no specific timing instructions. Add five to ten minutes with each subsequent application until an appropriate timing is reached (depending on harshness of ingredients):

astringents —10 to 20 minutes
masks —20 to 40 minutes
others —your own discretion

254

Whenever possible, apply cosmetics by patting on with fingertips. Otherwise, use pure absorbent cotton. In the case of masks, a brush may be called for. Use a soft paint brush or shaving brush with natural bristles, otherwise, apply with fingertips.

Opening Pores. Soak washcloth in very hot water, wring out and apply to area.

Closing Pores. After ingredients have been washed from face, remove remaining particles with warm washcloth. Splash face with cool, then cold water. Those sensitive to chlorine should splash spring water on the face, and apply cubes of ice made from drinking water.

EYE CARE

Puffiness. Steep 2 tea bags in boiling water and cool slightly. Or fill 2 homemade cheesecloth bags with a thick slice of peeled raw potato. Dab ½ teaspoon warm olive oil around eyes and on eyelids. Cover each eye with lukewarm tea bag or raw potato slice for 10 minutes. Gently rinse and pat dry.

FACIAL CARE

Masks. Masks are made for cleaning, moisturizing, and toning skin. The efficiency of using blanched almonds and oatmeal has been tested. However, for those sensitive to nuts and grains, it is suggested that the patient prepare her own meal with peanuts, soy beans, sunflower seed, potato meal, millet meal, or any meal that can be tolerated.

Almond mask: Blend 2 ounces blanched almonds to the consistency of grated cheese. Add a few drops of water, if necessary. Yield ½ cup. Follow application method above.

Avocado mask: Beat together 1 tablespoon ripe avocado and a few drops of lemon juice. Apply to freshly scrubbed face and throat. Leave on 30 minutes; rinse with warm, then cool water.

Milk of Magnesia mask: Apply plain milk of magnesia over face and neck, as above.

Oatmeal mask: Blend 1 cup of oatmeal until powdery. Yields ¾ cup powdered meal. Add a few drops of water. Use application method above.

Yeast mask: Mix together 1 tablespoon powdered Brewer's yeast, and 3 tablespoons milk, and apply to clean face and neck. Allow mixture to dry on skin 15 to 30 minutes as required. Do not speak or use facial muscles in any way until the mask has fully dried. Loosen by steaming slightly with washcloth dipped in warm water. Gently rub face and neck to remove all traces of the mask. If you have dry skin, apply a thin film of salad oil and blot away any excess. *Warning:* Avoid if you are yeast sensitive.

Another method of cleaning the face is to steam the face with hot towels which have been dampened in a solution of vinegar and 1 quart of water. Wipe off layers of dead skin.

Astringents. Lemon juice: Dilute to proper strength for complexion.

Cucumber juice: wash, dry, and cut up ½ unpeeled cucumber; liquefy in blender or juicer; heat but do not boil. Strain through a mesh cloth. Refrigerate leftover supply.

Vinegar: blend until smooth ½ cup water and 1 teaspoon cream of tartar; add ¼ cup white wine vinegar; shake well.

Lettuce: Put lettuce in a blender and strain the juice through a cheesecloth, or put it in a juicer and make lettuce juice. Use the juice as an astringent; the enzymes will remove the oil from the face.

Cleansers. Combine 2 teaspoons almond meal (see masks above) and 3 teaspoons whole milk. Apply smoothly to wet, clean face. Remove. Wash face, close pores.

Combine 2 tablespoons ground oatmeal and enough hot water to make a spreadable paste. Smooth on gently. When paste has dried, remove, wash face, close pores, and apply an astringent.

For a deep-pore cleanser, mash 1 fresh, peeled tomato and add enough almond meal or substitute to make paste.

Clean Your Face without Soap or Cream. Wash your face and neck with olive and coconut oil. Then make a little lather in your hands with oatmeal flour and use it as a "scrub" to remove the oil, finishing with a sponge-off under running water. This leaves your skin marvelously soft. Rinse with cool milk if tolerated, otherwise water.

Conditioners. Blend 1½ teaspoons fresh strawberry juice and 2 teaspoons butter. Apply smoothly and leave on for 15 minutes. Remove with soap and water, close pores.

Beat 1 egg until stiff; add 1 teaspoon honey, 1 teaspoon lemon juice. Mix, apply to face with fingertips. Remove when hardened. Wash face, close pores.

Moisturizers. Combine 1 teaspoon honey, 1 tablespoon strong herb tea and 1 tablespoon yogurt. Apply smoothly, remove, wash face, close pores.

Combine 1 teaspoon mayonnaise and 1 egg yolk. Apply with soft brush. Remove. Wash face, close pores.

Oily Skin Tonic. Wash face. Pat with strained juice of tomato, cucumber, or orange. Rinse with cool water, or rub face with slice of fresh tomato, cucumber, or orange.

Facial Rinse. Combine ¼ cup fresh parsley, 1 teaspoon dried mint leaves and 1 cup boiling water. Steep for 35 to 40 minutes. Strain and bottle. Use rinse each time you wash your face.

Softeners. Combine 1 tablespoon honey and 1 tablespoon molasses. Pat on face. Wash, close pores.

Mix 1 tablespoon honey, 1 tablespoon sour cream. Add enough cornstarch, potato, or arrowroot starch to make a thin paste. Apply. Remove, wash face, close pores.

Tightener. In blender, puree 1 small, fresh, peeled peach. Beat to a froth 1 egg white. Combine ingredients and apply smoothly. Remove, wash face, close pores.

HAIR CARE

All-purpose Treatment and Shampoo. Beat to a froth 2 egg yolks and 2 teaspoons almond oil. Massage into scalp and spread through hair. Leave on until it stiffens, at least 1 hour—the longer, the better. Rinse thoroughly with water only. This treatment is highly recommended. Some individuals have given up all other hair care after a year of this treatment. If you cannot use almond oil, substitute an oil that can be tolerated.

Combs and Brushes. Avoid plastic combs; metal ones and wooden ones are available at health food stores. Use a wooden handled, natural bristle hair brush.

Conditioner. Beat 1 egg yolk well. Add ½ cup yogurt and continue to beat well. After shampooing hair, gently comb the mixture through the hair and let stand for 20 to 30 minutes. Rinse thoroughly with warm water.

Conditioner for Dry Hair. Blend ⅓ peeled ripe avocado and ⅓ cup mayonnaise. Massage into scalp and work through hair. Rinse and shampoo.

Dandruff Treatments. Combine ½ cup apple cider vinegar and ½ cup water. Apply directly to the scalp a few times a week before shampooing.

Rinse hair with a solution of Zephiran 1:750 (½ teaspoon to 1 cup water). Zephiran may also be used as a general disinfectant.

Dry Hair Treatment. Gently massage 2 tablespoons mayonnaise into the hair. Rinse, shampoo.

Hairdryer. Avoid plastic. Find an old-style metal dryer.

Hair Spray (nonchemical). Mix ⅛ teaspoon powdered gelatin in ⅙ cup cool water. Heat in top of double boiler, stirring to dissolve. Transfer into a spray atomizer. Store supply in refrigerator. Heat before use.

For an emergency solution to flyaway hair, pat fresh lemon juice on difficult-to-maintain areas; or make your own lemon hair spray. Chop 1 whole lemon and cover with hot water, bring to boil, and boil down until half the original quantity of water remains. Cool. Squeeze lemon and liquid through thin cloth or cheesecloth strainer. If too thick, add water and mix well. Refrigerate in pump valve dispenser (such as is used for washing windows.)

Rinses. Combine ½ cup strained lemon juice and 1 cup distilled water. Shake well and comb thoroughly through hair after shampooing.

For oily hair: Diluted vinegar rinsed through hair, followed by clear water.

For blondes: Steep 2 tablespoons camomile in 2 cups fast-boiling water for 10 minutes. Cool and strain through unbleached muslin. Use as rinse after washing hair.

For brunettes: Steep 2 teaspoons dried rosemary in 2 cups fast-boiling water for 10 minutes. Use as rinse after washing hair.

Setting Lotions. Mix ½ cup warm water and 6 teaspoons superfine sugar—beet or cane if tolerated. Apply while warm to set curls.

Shampoos. See above: All-purpose Treatment and Shampoo.

Amino Pon is available at beauty shops. For distributors write: Redken Laboratories, Canoga Park, California 91303. The pure castile shampoo by Almay does not have a petroleum base. Some have been able to tolerate it. Johnson's Baby Shampoo can be tolerated by some. Others can tolerate Arex or Marcelle, unscented.

Homemade shampoo: Place the remains of face soaps in a jar with enough spring water to cover. After soaking for a few days, run through a blender, first at low speed, then at high. Reblend shampoo each time before use to prevent congealing. Optional for those who tolerate eggs: Add an egg for each shampoo. A pure castile soap is good for this mixture.

Beat together 1 egg and 1 pint cool water. Work into the hair thoroughly. Rinse well with lukewarm water. For last rinse, add one tablespoon lemon juice to 1 pint of water.

MAKEUP

Eyebrow Pencil. Charcoal from a wood fire works well for some who can tolerate nothing else. Test carefully. Keep in metal or china pillbox.

Face Cream. Some beauty consultants recommend mayonnaise as a face cream. Make your own; any tolerated oil can be used. Those allergic to eggs can try an eggless mayonnaise (see page 302).

Here is a recipe for face cream or body lotion that really does the trick. However, in making it one must experiment, since there are many variables, such as room temperature of the oil or speed of the blender. Mix well 1 ounce oil and 1 teaspoon acacia (gum arabic) in blender. When firm, add 1 ounce water. The thicker the oil, the more acacia is needed. Whip until frothy and emulsified.

Face Powder. For face powder, brown arrowroot starch in a dry skillet over low heat. It will change color evenly as you stir it. Continue stirring until the desired shade is obtained. It takes about 35 minutes to produce a light ivory shade. The pressed form of face powder by Marcelle is tolerated by a few very sensitive people.

A recipe for oatmeal face powder: Crush organic rolled oats in a tea strainer or flour sifter until it becomes a fine powder. In the palm of your hand make a paste of a pinch of oat powder and a few drops of water. Rub this paste briskly over the face and neck. When it dries, brush off the residue. The face will have a lovely matte finish.

Lipstick. To date, we have found no pure product substitute.

BODY CARE

Bath Powder or Dusting Powder. Any tolerated starch such as arrowroot, or tapioca, is effective.

Bath Water. For chlorine-sensitive persons, a few crystals of sodium thiosulphate changes chlorine to chloride.

Bathing. Long luxurious baths are not recommended. Some gynecologists warn that baths deplete your skin of oils and hormones. Women over thirty-five should avoid baths in favor of no more than three short showers a week. Clean yourself frequently with short sponge baths.

Take 1 bar pure castile soap, 1 quart water, ¼ cup olive oil and simmer together until soap is completely melted. Cool. Use in place of soap for shower or tub bath. Excellent for dry skin.

Body Brush. The loofah plant, available at health food stores, makes a good body brush. Ask for Spa Genuine Loofa by Schroeder and Tremayne, Inc., or contact Kennedy Natural Food Store (see page 329).

Deodorant. The best deodorants are natural dark green plants particularly parsley and comfrey. When available in quantity, juice them and store them as ice cubes. Drink the juice alone or, to make it more palatable, mix with another juice.

Blend in the blender ½ cup baking soda and ½ cup arrowroot starch. An effective deodorant and excellent powder for your whole body. Those sensitive to arrowroot starch should substitute another kind.

Five-day deodorant pads can be used by some who are quite sensitive. Others can use plain baking soda or the alkali salt mixture of ⅔ soda bicarbonate and ⅓ potassium bicarbonate.

For a deodorant anti-perspirant, Dr. Randolph recommends that a druggist be asked to make the following: aluminum chloride 4 gm. and water to make 100cc. or, especially if you cannot tolerate aluminum, oxyquinoline sulfate 1 gm. and rose water to make 500cc. Either should be tried on a small area to test for individual tolerance.

Herb Baths. Baths are not recommended. However, if you occasionally feel you need one to relax, try an herb bath.

Put ½ handful dry mint, thyme, and rosemary, the peel of one lemon, the peel of one orange, and rose petals in the toe of a stocking or tie up in cheesecloth. Omit anything you cannot tolerate, anything you are sensitive to. Draw very hot bath water; let herb bag steep in the tub until water cools to proper temperature.

Rough Skin. Rub tomato slice on elbows and heels. The tannic acid content softens rough skin. Avocado is also good for elbows, heels, and even for the face.

Skin Oil. Use tolerated vegetable or fruit oil for face and body lubrication after bath. Coconut oil, almond oil, and apricot oil seem to be the most effective. Pat skin partially dry, apply oil to skin, rub in with the remaining moisture, and allow to dry. This is a good foundation for face powder if allowed to dry for 15 minutes.

Soap. If not available at health food stores, Nature Born Oatmeal and Bran complexion soaps can be ordered from Anne Carpenter Cosmetics, Inc., Weston, Vermont, 05161. Conte castile soap is available in drug stores, and is not perfumed. It is made with olive oil and is especially good for dry skin.

Sunburn Preparations. Sunbathing is not recommended for anyone subject to allergies. However, since the sun cannot always be avoided, here are a few treatments to protect skin exposed or overexposed to the sun:

Thoroughly mix 1 cup buttermilk and strained juice of 2 fresh tomatoes. Apply to the affected area. Rinse in shower. To relieve sunburn, make a paste of ½ cup baking soda, a pinch of salt, and a few drops of water. Spread gently over affected area. Rinse in tepid bath when paste dries. Apple cider vinegar can also be applied for sunburn relief.

Teeth. The safest way to clean teeth for those most sensitive to chemicals is with pure baking soda, pure sea salt, or a combination of the two. Sensodyne toothpaste is corn-free and can be tolerated by some people who cannot use other toothpastes.

Formula for tooth powder: In a blender, whip until pulverized, ¾ cup of salt. Add ½ pound baking soda. Blend until reduced to a very fine powder. Optional, add *one* herb for flavoring: cassia, or a mint.

CHAPTER 29

Travel

With PROPER clinical management of allergies to foods, drugs, and chemicals, even the most severely affected individuals improve and can return to a relatively normal life style, including traveling. Moreover, with enough planning and ingenuity, travel can be managed and enjoyed even during the most acute allergic stage, if you are willing to accept the challenge. This chapter includes information gathered from many sensitive people who did just that.[1]

Very few persons will have to take into account all these suggestions, but the help is here if you need it. For those of you who are interested in prevention, you will find that you will be able to follow many of these procedures with very little, if any, extra cost and still be able to enjoy a healthier environment during your travels.

In the broadest sense "travel" is any excursion that takes you away from home. The first circle is defined by the daily traveling of the family: getting to and from work, grocery shopping, doctor's visits, chauffeuring children to commitments. A larger compass would include emergency or necessary out-of-town trips—weddings, funerals, graduations. An enlarging series of ventures implies pleasure jaunts, retreats to mountain hideaways, and vacations.

AUTO TRAVEL

Air Conditioning. Automobile air conditioners installed at the factory often have a fixed intake of outside air. If so, it is preferable to have a service station install the recirculating type to prevent road and engine fumes from coming through vents.

Whenever you are planning to use the air conditioner in your car, follow the procedures as outlined:

1. Open all the windows and doors to let the car air out as long as possible before starting the motor.

2. Close the windows, start the motor, and begin to drive before reopening the windows and before turning on the air conditioner. This

261

is important in order to avoid fumes which accumulate from starting the motor.

3. After the car is in motion, drive with the windows open and the air conditioning on for five or ten minutes in order to allow the mold that has gathered in the air conditioner overnight to be dispersed by the wind.

4. Now close all the windows again.

5. Whenever there is heavy pollution, or whenever you are in very heavy traffic, keep your air conditioner on maximum cool even if it is necessary to wear a sweater and to cover your legs with a blanket. The force of the air conditioning helps keep the fumes from entering the car.

Air Filter. Keep the air filter clean. Change it often. Any competent mechanic will be able to find your air filter, which is located in the middle of your engine.

Air the Car. Clean and air the car several times a day when traveling. By leaving the main road, you can park and open the doors to let in fresh air. If there is a breeze, park on the upwind side so fumes from the road blow away from you.

Auto Choice. A car which is at least two years old will have a relatively seasoned plastic interior. The nonexistent perfect car would not have a plastic interior (check Mercedes and Lincoln). It would be tightly constructed to prevent its own exhaust fumes from backing into the engine. The air conditioner would have recirculating air (not "fresh" air intake from roadways), and the heater would be free of plastic parts. This car would have power windows enabling speedy closing of all the windows when you are passing a freshly tarred or similarly toxic area. After emerging from pollution, you could quickly open all the windows to clear out the fumes that had seeped into the car. The car would have heavy cotton seat covers, securely anchored and yet removable for laundering, no mothproofed or synthetic carpets, or rubber mats.

Since there is no perfect car, settle for second best—meaning, whatever you can tolerate. Shop around and subject cars to the sniff test.

Cleaning. Soap-and-water scrubbing followed by vinegar rinsing will help (a little) to get rid of powerful smells which fuse themselves into the plastic and/or leather.

Clothing. When clothes are taken from a suitcase, they should be aired by placing them on a shower rod either with the bathroom exhaust fan running or by using an air purifier. Plan to travel in comfortable clothing that you know will not cause problems.

Exhaust. Taking the back roads (although the long way around) often makes the difference between a pleasant trip and a headache. If the main problem is from exhaust fumes, avoid rush hour traffic; nighttime travel is preferable.

Do not reverse your car with windows or vents open; exhaust fumes will pour inside. Avoid driving behind buses or trucks; get into the other lane. Turn air conditioning on to recirculate air (even in the winter); the increased pressure inside will help to keep out fumes.

Develop new driving habits. Do not follow too closely behind the car ahead of you. If a truck is in front of you, and you are on a four- or six-lane highway, change lanes and either pass the truck, if he is going slowly, or slow down and let him get farther ahead of you.

Be aware of red lights. When you see a red light ahead, slow down, approaching it slowly so that it will have time to change. If it is still red when you reach the intersection, leave a couple of car lengths between you and the car in front of you. Then inch up very slowly toward that car so that the fumes that have gathered underneath your car will not become excessive.

If as you approach a traffic light it is green, move a little faster so that you can get through the green light. In other words, pace yourself reasonably without tying up traffic at an intersection, so you will not inhale your car's exhaust fumes or those of other cars.

For the same reason, whenever possible, avoid letting your motor idle. If you are waiting for someone to enter or leave the car, turn off the motor.

Filters. Plug-in car charcoal filters, when obtainable, help to absorb plastic vapors as well as exhaust fumes. A car filter that plugs into the cigarette lighter can be purchased. It contains activated charcoal and Purafil and is particularly helpful when driving in heavily polluted areas.[2]

From the same concern you can inquire about a portable purse-size filter, the size and shape of an eight-ounce bottle of juice with a bamboo mouthpiece. It is called "the junior sized personal air depollution unit." Your lungs supply the fan.

Although the most effective filtering unit is made of nylon, for those sensitive to nylon a linen, silk, or cotton filter can be substituted. This kind of portable filter requires a prescription from your physician.

Because it is possible that a user could inhale charcoal and thereby become allergic to it, this filter should be saved for emergency situations, for example, in a car, if the electric filter is not working.

A purse-size filter can be made by filling an oblong bag of heavy cotton with activated charcoal. Charcoal is most often made from coal but it is also made from coconut and other shells. If one experiences a dryness in the nasal passages from breathing through charcoal, it can be lessened by placing a layer of wool (if tolerated) between the charcoal and the cotton covering. A washable outer case is desirable. To lengthen the usefulness of the filter, store it when not in use in a metal container such as a Band-aid box.

Gas and Oil. RPM or Quaker State oil are relatively odor-free for normal operation. Be sure to use unleaded gasoline.

Heater. Do not use the heater except when absolutely necessary, because it draws in fumes from the engine and the road. Dress warmly. The Audi has a heater fan for intake air located so that it can be covered with a fine mesh screen containing activated charcoal, and some people can use this heater without problems.

Highways. When traveling on superhighways there are certain precautions and practices which aid the driver. Determine from which direction the wind is blowing and, if traffic conditions permit, drive so that the wind will carry exhaust fumes away from the driver. When on a stretch of road with no cars nearby, open the windows and revitalize the interior air. Observe the drift of smoke from diesel trucks and check tree leaves for an indicator of wind direction. Be aware of the exhaust pipe of the car ahead and stay far behind it.

Metal Carriers. It is advisable to carry lunches and extra clothing in metal boxes. Cardboard boxes and suitcases may give off vapors which soon permeate the closed-up space of a car interior. The metal Portafile box is excellent for this purpose.

Overcoming Vinyl Interiors. Cars two years old or older usually give fewer problems because the vinyl has aged. Body heat on vinyl seats produces head pressure and drowsiness as well as other physical and mental symptoms that make driving uncomfortable and even dangerous. Sensitive persons should sit on blankets or towels.

Make seat covers from old cotton mattress pads covered with untreated cotton to keep down fumes from heat, sun, or the human body. Denim and sailcloth make good seat covers. The most efficient seat covers can be made from cotton (preferably denim) lined with the barrier cloth discussed in Chapter 26.

Barrier cloth lined with denim, or even alone, could be a good buffer to line the carpets of the car, if they cannot be removed. It would be even better to make a new carpet from cotton quilting lined with barrier cloth and with an attractive cotton fabric as its cover.

For some people leather seats are a good solution when they can be ordered. Shearling fleece seat covers are available in some catalogs.[3] Check on mothproofing and buy on approval.

Wash vinyl interiors with a strong solution of cider vinegar, rinse, and dry well. Repeat several times, particularly on new cars. If that doesn't help, try baking soda and water.

One very sensitive man found that the only way he could tolerate the vinyl interior of a car was to coat it with beeswax. This idea should be approached with great caution for the *very* sensitive, many of whom find beeswax intolerable.

This treatment does not refer to seat covers, just to the plastic (on dashboards, doors,) that cannot be covered with fabric. A film forms on the inside of car windows from the particles of plastic released from vinyl upholstery, which gives you an idea of how much plastic may be inhaled by the average passenger. This must be reduced by every possible means.

Suitcases. Avoid new luggage. Use sniff test before using old luggage. Even if suitcases are aired ahead of time, they still may cause trouble. Keep charcoal bags inside suitcases when not in use.

Travel Problem. If hydrocarbon combustion and tobacco smoke cause cerebral edema, consider the advisability of traveling with someone who understands the problem.

Travel Time. Early morning is preferable to afternoon. Sea or mountain air on one side of the car is helpful; tunnels, refineries, and agricultural sprays are hazardous. If traveling from a populated area to a less populated area, plan to leave when traffic is light.

Vapors. A car with a cool interior will give off less plastic vapor than a heated interior. This may mean driving with little or no use of the heater in the winter, and it certainly means using an air conditioner liberally in warm weather. In the summer when traveling by car, it is least toxic to travel in the middle of the night.

TRAIN TRAVEL

Diesel-powered cars on trains, even when empty, are smelly because the smoke blows back and down upon the cars. Passenger cars near the end of the train are least objectionable. Roomettes, although cheaper than compartments, are smaller and less airy. The affected individual should make a charcoal "gas mask," take his own food and his own bed linen and towels with name tags on them. Coaches should be considered only as a last resort.

BUS TRAVEL

Bus terminals in downtown urban centers mean traffic problems, but at least the bus exhaust is in the back. For those allergic to tobacco, a bus would not be advisable.

AIRLINE TRAVEL

Standing in line at an airport, where people are smoking or wearing heavy perfume is not a good idea. Use a charcoal filter or ask to be preboarded. You will be exposed to fumes as the plane idles, but if you have a pillow or a handkerchief containing activated charcoal or a purse-size filter, it is better to be preboarded so you can sit in one place and protect yourself by breathing into the filter. When making reservations, ask to speak with the supervisor and arrange for "Extra Care Code." The following is an account of what can be done, if the airline is approached properly.

When one patient was making reservations with United Airlines, she spoke to the supervisor, explained her problem, and asked to be allowed to wait in a small private room away from the smoke. A United supervisor took her to such a room where she waited until called. She was then allowed to board the plane before the other passengers. The supervisor introduced her to the stewardess and explained that she was traveling under "Extra Care Code."

On the flight, when she took oxygen, the stewardess warned nearby passengers not to smoke. On the return flight, by explaining what had been done for her on the earlier flight, she received the same good service plus more. Because the plane was not filled, the flight attendant kept the row of seats beside and behind her empty. United Airlines even granted her permission to carry on board a five-foot International Heater. (Permission must be asked in advance.) Whenever possible, try flying United Airlines because doctors have reported greater attention to health needs of their patients than from other airlines.

Nonstop flights are better than flights with intermediary stops, for obvious reasons.

Airports. Airports have their own special kinds of smog concentration, but once you are airborne, the travel time saved makes this mode of transportation desirable.*

Oxygen. A letter from the doctor describing the patient's reactions is useful. Airline officials and flight attendants have a profound respect for a green tank of oxygen with a prescription-type regulator.

HOTELS AND MOTELS

Bathroom. One with an extreme allergy should take his own soap and, upon arrival at the hotel or motel, use his soap and the hotel's

---

* See bibliography in *Human Ecology* for Dr. Theron Randolph's article on foreign travel.

towels to wash the bathroom tub, sink and floor. Then, if he cannot tolerate the room, he can sleep in the bathroom which has been made fairly free from excitants. One severely affected patient, anticipating such a problem, carried a cot in the trunk of the car. If necessary, remove the plastic shower curtain.

It is advisable to carry with you a bottle of Zephiran 1:750. Be sure it is aqueous Zephiran and not the tinctured kind. It can be used as a disinfectant to clear away the molds or the odors from the bathroom.

Linens. Take linens if there is a problem with treated cottons, synthetics, or detergents. Carry with you a sheet of barrier cloth. It may help to minimize the exposure of a treated mattress or a foam mattress.

Maid Service. Ask that no maid service be given during the stay of an acutely allergic individual.

Pick Your Hotel Wisely. By calling ahead of arrival, you can ascertain if a motel or hotel will be suitable. Avoid community hazards such as chemical plants, refineries, airports. Pick a motel off the highway with small parking squares in front of units. Lawns and gardens around swimming pools probably mean insect repellent and fertilizers. Fans blowing across running water carry chlorine fumes.

The Hyatt-Regency chain of hotels, based in Atlanta, has announced a new policy designed to accommodate nonsmokers and sensitive persons. Each Hyatt-Regency will set aside separate floors where smoking will be prohibited. Guests will be asked about smoking preferences and assigned accordingly. In addition, Hyatt-Regency dining rooms have separate no-smoking sections.

When checking with the management, you should consider the following items: electric heat, bathrooms with exhaust fans, kitchenettes with electric stoves and refrigerators. When possible ask them to reserve a room on the second-floor level of a motel; the higher, the better, in a hotel. If there are fans which blow air into the room from other parts of the motel, ask to have them turned off to avoid a neighbor's perfumes and smoke.

Request a room that has not been exterminated recently, and has no air freshener. Ask them to open the windows, if possible, to air the room before your arrival time. Try to get a room with a minimum of floor covering.

Ask if they have recently painted the room or even the halls or any other room on that floor. If they have done so recently or are planning to do so during your stay, ask that a room be reserved on a different floor where there will be no paint fumes. If you have a choice, reserve a room in an older section of the hotel which has not recently been decorated.

When checking in, ask to inspect your room. Explain your problem.

Test the room for ten or twenty minutes before unpacking or disturbing it. Indicate your intention to the desk clerk and the bellman. Whenever possible select a room that is farthest from the mainstream of traffic.

Be pleasant but firm. A little generous tipping goes a long way. The service people in a hotel are more willing to cooperate when their efforts are rewarded with pleasantness and honesty.

You may find in some hotels that the first, second, or third room you go to is not acceptable, but another will suffice. If, however, it is hopeless, try to find accommodations in another hotel or motel.

TRAVEL TRAILERS

To solve the overnighting problem, many allergic persons are turning to recreational vehicles. Some are able to use campers and motor homes successfully, but this is not a solution for those who react strongly to automobile fumes, for it is the equivalent of having a gasoline motor in your bedroom.

For these people, the best results will probably be obtained with a travel trailer, which is towed by a separate car.

In choosing such a trailer, watch for the following points:

Air Conditioning. Trailer air conditioning is essential for the chemically sensitive, for exposure to outdoor contaminants is unavoidable in a trailer park. This often means keeping the trailer closed and air-conditioned for comfortable sleeping. Most trailers can be equipped with ceiling air-conditioning units installed by the dealer.

Avoid Secondhand Trailers. It is better to buy a new trailer; it will air out quickly. Most secondhand trailers have been sprayed with pesticides and have been contaminated by use of bottled gas.

Electricity. Make sure all appliances will operate electrically, substituting for gas where necessary. Most trailer refrigerators operate on either electricity or gas. This is sometimes true of water heaters, although electric ones are available. Electric hot plates, crock pots, and ovens will usually meet cooking needs.

Heating. Combination window units which provide heat and air conditioning are available. (Be careful to have such a unit installed where it will not disturb weight distribution in the trailer and create handling problems.) Old-fashioned electrical space heaters, built before the advent of plastic-coated wiring, are probably the most successful means of heating a trailer. *Be sure to check the filter.*

Plastics. Make sure that walls and cabinets are wood and that the interior contains a minimum of plastic. Bathrooms are always constructed of plastic but these can be shut off to keep fumes from the sleeping area.

Remove all foam rubber mattresses and cushions and substitute tolerable materials. If this is not possible, cover foam cushions with heavy-duty aluminum foil, followed by several layers of tolerated fabric (usually well-washed cotton material). If barrier cloth can be tolerated, you may need only one layer.

Power Supply. For full electrical operation, a trailer park will have to be capable of supplying you with 50-amp service. This may be an occasional problem, but well-known parks are nearly always able to meet these needs.

MISCELLANEOUS TRAVEL TIPS

Even during the acute stage of your allergy, if you maintain your diet and keep your bedroom environment relatively free, you can tolerate the added exposure you will receive while traveling. The following checklist may be of help.

Items to Take:
1. Four food lists, one for each of the following types of food: frozen, fresh, bottled, packaged
2. Equipment for cooking
3. Linens (napkins, dishtowels, dish cloths, sheets, blankets) for those who cannot tolerate synthetics, detergents, or bleach
4. Clothes
5. Cot (for those who cannot tolerate mattresses)
6. Soap, shampoo, and other special needs not easily obtainable
7. Travel kit: perhaps a strong tote bag, one quart of water, a bottle of Zephiran, small quantity of medication, one-day food supply, charcoal filter, oxygen equipment, an extra package of protein (to anticipate being stranded without food for some time)

Advance Arrangements to Be Made. When possible, enlist the aid of someone located in the area where you will be visiting. Otherwise, the yellow pages can help locate the following:
1. Water supply
2. Health food store
3. Oxygen supply (the regulator for the "D" & "E" tanks fits the "D" & "E" tanks of all companies)
4. Sleeping accommodations
5. Cooking facilities
6. Freezer space (at a private home, freezer locker, church refrigerator or butcher shop)

Packaging Food. Food may be the biggest problem, especially if organic food is needed and it has not been possible to locate a local source of food.

Several days before your trip, purchase sturdy special boxes 10½" × 10½" × 36" available from dry ice distributors. This allows you time to measure the space needed for food and purchase more boxes if necessary. The distributors can advise you on the amount of dry ice needed. Do not skimp; it's better to waste dry ice than have food spoilage.

Buy the dry ice at the last possible minute. The bags of frozen food must go directly from the freezer to the boxes with the dry ice and be sealed immediately. Do not allow any time for the slightest thaw.

Do not rely on dry ice for precooked food for more than thirty-six to forty-eight hours. It is safer to take frozen, uncooked food, removing it to a refrigerator when the ice evaporates and cooking it within two or three days after it thaws.

Do not pack fresh food with frozen food.

Canned Ice. This, when frozen solid overnight in the freezer compartment, takes the place of ice, with no drip and no mess; it is reusable. Canned ice can be used for fresh foods that have to be kept cold. If enough cans have been frozen solid and if your frozen food is in large pieces (such as huge roasts), and if you are not traveling too far, canned ice will keep frozen foods from thawing. It is not always available in metal containers. You may have to order by mail.[4]

While the special boxes purchased at dry ice distributors are satisfactory, cardboard boxes must be carefully examined to be sure they have not been exposed to insecticides. Cardboard retains the odor of insecticides indefinitely; the glue used in its manufacture is toxic. Another shortcoming of cardboard boxes is that you must keep them in the car; you cannot put them into the trunk where the food will be permeated with the odors of tires and fumes from the automobile.

It is advisable to buy galvanized cans (such as garbage cans in various sizes) in which food can be sealed. These can be placed in the trunk of the car.

A similarly safe storage place is an old-fashioned milk can. These can be purchased at auctions or at secondhand stores in rural districts. Just be sure they are not rancid from milk or moldy from dampness.

Wrap all precooked food in meal-size packages. On the label, write the contents of the package with the day of the week and the date the food is to be eaten. The menu should be planned for each day of the trip including every little detail such as salt and herbs. In this way no item will be overlooked.

Much of the foregoing may seem overpowering and discouraging. Keep in mind that extreme caution is needed only by very severe cases in their most acute stages. You can select the precautions you must take.

One patient, who once had to carry everything, including her heater, cot, bedding, and food, now reports that she travels like anyone else, maintaining her diet as best she can, but breaking it when she cannot avoid doing so. When she gets home, she returns to her diet of "organic foods" and the comparatively pure environment of her home.

CHAPTER 30

Mental Attitude

To REMAIN mentally healthy in spite of physical discomfort and medical problems takes concentration and will power. Yet, it is of paramount importance because so much of your future well being depends on it.

Many patients, normally free from depression, have experienced a state of depression when exposed to certain chemical excitants. Frequently, this causes members of the family and even the family physician to suspect that the condition is psychosomatic.

Similarly, after the allergens have been physically purged, the mental state returns to normal. Since this has happened with many allergic reactors, the patient with this problem should accept the word of the doctor who has diagnosed his particular case of depression as chemical reaction. However, he must avoid applying this interpretation to other persons who suffer from depression.

It is also entirely possible for a person to be allergic and have, in addition, a completely unrelated emotional problem. Diagnosing depression—or undue elation—as induced by toxic stresses is one of the toughest challenges that a clinical ecologist faces. A patient cannot judge this for himself; he can assume nothing. This chapter has been prepared primarily for those whose emotional reactions are interrelated with a chemical reaction.

A positive mental attitude is important. Even when the food or chemical excitant is a prime factor in depression, there is no purpose in allowing yourself to wallow in self-pity. Just as you would take action to gain physical relief, so you must force yourself to do something about your mental state. Experience has shown that the physical reaction can be purged more quickly than the emotional factor. Granted, the very condition of depression frequently robs you of your initiative, your fight, your determination. You should seek help from others with the same problem.[1] See Chapter 1 for details about this organization, named HEAL.

In order to be of help to one another, you must understand that the proper mental attitude should be of concern to all, not just those with health problems.

272

During the period of testing, and later of adjusting to one's environment, seeing friends often becomes a source of harassment, rather than pleasure. Many have been unable to visit homes of parents and friends who heat with gas or use gas stoves.

The constant need for explanation and excuses to the "nonbeliever" causes frustration, embarrassment, and despair. In the beginning, it may seem a losing battle to try to maintain the status quo. Until the adjustment has been made, search out others who share this problem. When your health has improved, you can always return to former friends; you will be richer by having made new ones.

Visit the homes of other patients. Here you will find a compatible environment and tolerable food. Avoid one pitfall: making the visit a rehash of symptoms, a discussion of problems. After the initial discovery of mutual complaints, the subject should be dropped.

When you are forced to change your food habits, your social habits, your home environment, and your wearing apparel, is it any wonder that you tend to become too absorbed in yourself? You must avoid the trap of self-absorption. How? By becoming absorbed in others—as well as yourself—by an exchange of ideas.

Fight illness with what might be called the "buddy system." If you are one who reacts to excitants by experiencing depression, it is important to have someone to help you. Because problems do not always conform to the office hours of professionals, you must sometimes turn to the nonprofessional. Friends and relatives seldom can be of any real help because they cannot fully understand what they have not experienced—they tend to aggravate the condition by suggesting it is all in the mind.

Choose a buddy from the organization HEAL. By prior arrangement, when you call and in tears say, "Make me laugh," your buddy will immediately understand. "Make me laugh" has been selected as the password, because it eloquently expresses the basis of the person-to-person "buddy therapy." Of all the bromides applicable to patients, probably the most useful is, "laughter is the best medicine."

When it is your turn to help, be sympathetic and understanding, but keep leading the subject away from the trouble and the problem. It has been tested and it works. Strangely enough, it often does not really matter much what you say as long as you laugh and feel for each other. Those are the two most important ingredients. Patients have often helped each other when both of them were having reactions and suffering from mental confusion as well as depression. Laughter acts as an emotional catharsis and seems to be to the psyche what salts or enemas are to the body. We urge you to try it.

Another by-product of the buddy plan is the sharing of physical exercise. It is well known that physical exercise is important to the patient; an easing of symptoms has been experienced as a result of it. Yet you might resent someone telling you to exercise your weary, painful muscles unless the suggestion comes from a fellow sufferer. Two members separated by a great distance make a daily phone call to check with each other about their exercises. Here again, first consult your physician about the proper exercise for you and your condition.

It is unfortunate that space prevents us from sharing some amusing experiences. In the interest of expediency, we have written our book in a serious rather than a light vein. However, this should not set the pattern for your mental attitude. You should share your funny experiences with other members. The humorous aspect of your problem should be looked at and laughed at to lighten the mood. As one patient has said, "I laugh about it so I won't cry."

That very often is the best solution. However, the value of a good cry with all stops pulled out should not be underestimated. A good cry at home with friends will prevent you from deadening your relationships by constant complaining. If you can honestly face the fact that your friends and relatives frequently receive the brunt of the anger and frustration caused by your problems, you can learn to direct the irritation elsewhere.

Many patients have found that their reactions tend to be more severe when chemical exposure is compounded by emotional stress. If you feel overwhelmed by your problems, give in to the frustration; let the frustation take over, so that you can pound it out into a pillow. If you're angry, pound a mattress.

Exercises combined with breathing techniques to release emotional tension do help. (Many patients have found that exercise in any form is helpful, particularly yoga exercises which teach proper breathing. As always, check first with your doctor before attempting any form of exercise.) Any kind of self-relaxation exercise is helpful. Many patients have learned to reduce their allergic reactions by listening to a cassette tape entitled *Self-relaxation* (send $9.00 to Synesthetics Inc., Producer and Distributor, Box 254, Cos Cob, Connecticut 06807).

Some patients have found the following exercise helpful: Walk around the room stamping with equal force on the heels and balls of your feet; accompany each stamping motion with a movement of clenched fists pounding downward as if striking straight down into the floor. Coordinate these movements with a loud, resounding exhale that sounds like "Hah." After circling the room three or four times, change the foot and leg movement by kicking outward into space as if you were trying to kick your heel into something suspended two or three feet in the air. Coordinate this movement with a thrust of your fists at the same imaginary object, using the same loud exhaling sound of "Hah."

As with any exercise, begin slowly, working only five minutes, and with each exposure gradually increase the length of time.

This exercise is particularly effective after driving through heavy traffic. It will help clear the lungs and increase the circulation in the extremities. It has proved especially helpful for patients who do not have arthritis, but react to certain chemicals with arthriticlike pains.

A healthy mental attitude about food is as important as the attitude about exercise. Stop thinking of yourself as deprived. This should be the number one rule for any kind of diet. Avoid talking about the difficulties and hardships of dieting.

"Regarding giving up favorite foods, or trying new ones," says Dr. Karl Humiston, "the main problems come when focusing on your thoughts rather than your senses. The more you *think about* trying unfamiliar food, or being without familiar ones, the more upset you can become.

"Your body has the answer, when you turn your thoughts there. Lie down, or sit with your feet flat, with your eyes closed. Experience, or think about, what you are facing in today's eating.

"Locate where your body is responding to the experience, where you can find any physical sensation—tightness, heaviness, warmth, shaking, or anything.

"Focus on that location as long as the feeling is there, letting your attention go to your thoughts as often as it wants, or bringing it back to the place in your body that's feeling something at the moment.

"Thoughts can be intolerable. The body feelings you will get from this method can *always* be tolerated—if you stay with them as long as they are there.

"Further, in some mysterious way, locating your body sensations in this way, puts you in touch with your inner energy flow, leading to insights and awarenesses, more energy, and greater enjoyment of your new way of eating."

In an interview, Dr. Michael Schachter mentioned his concern that chemically sensitive patients, unless guided properly, might become food faddists because of their preoccupation with diet.[2] He believes that once the patient develops a diet he can live with he should stop analyzing it, stop thinking in terms of "Now I'm eating fats, now I'm eating protein, now I'm eating carbohydrates." He should simply eat and enjoy it.

Dr. Schachter feels that it is important for the patient to avoid thinking in terms of being deprived but rather to think of it as a learning experience. He should regard it as an opportunity to explore and experiment, to increase and widen the range of foods possible.

WILLINGNESS TO BREAK OUT OF AN OLD LIFE STYLE

Frankly, you may not be able to continue your life as before; you may have to change jobs, residence, and recreational habits. This does not mean you have to crawl into the house and stay there. Once you accept chemical intolerances and deal with the resulting frustrations, an enjoyable life style is possible if you are willing to be flexible and creatively seek positive alternatives.

Help is available from surprising sources. An outgrowth of the so-called "hippie movement" has been a renewed interest in natural living and crafts. Shops that were once confined to Greenwich Village now abound in most large cities or near colleges; they are stacked with books about natural living. Typical offerings include *Mother Earth News* and *The Whole Earth Catalogue*. There, you can learn anything from how to butcher a hog to making a rope bed. The bulletin boards at health food stores list persons who are working with various extinct crafts. Many larger cities have a "Switchboard" (the actual name; call Information for the number).

While Switchboard was set up for young people, it is a good source of information on where to buy pure items. Underground newspapers also present useful ideas for natural living and carry ads for goods and services.

Look to the past for ideas to build your future. Historical societies are often helpful. The staff usually delights in helping find a source for pure items or a historical way of doing things. Your public librarian should be asked for help in locating a historical society or in finding information. Almost all libraries can borrow books from larger libraries all around the country. Consumer services columns in local newspapers can help locate items for you.

Becoming flexible may mean that you should begin to haunt charity thrift shops. What good are the best shops, even if you can afford them, if they cannot offer a product you can tolerate? It may mean seeking recreation outdoors instead of in nightclubs and restaurants, the mountains instead of exciting cities, hobbies or crafts instead of smoke-filled meetings.

Living with multiple allergies is not dull and it need not be depressing. Again, it all depends on your mental attitude and willingness to try something new.

PART VI

Cookbook for the Allergic Person

Introduction

REASONS FOR AVOIDING SUGAR *

Turn your back on sugar. Sugar in any form (including raw, turbanado, brown, beet, cane, maple, date, etc.) is strongly advised against in any good nutrition program, especially in the case of the allergic patient. According to Dr. Warren Levin, the four most important reasons for this prohibition are:

Blood Sugar Levels. Control of blood sugar (glucose) levels is the result of an exquisitely balanced mechanism in the healthy body, under the influence of the combined neuro-endocrine (brain-gland) systems. This machinery was *not* designed to cope with sudden, rapid, great changes in sugar levels. The total sugar circulating in the blood of the average person is approximately two teaspoons. One piece of apple pie à la mode contains *eighteen* teaspoons! Such severe disruptions in the body's equilibrium is a severe *stress*. This, in particular, overworks the adrenal gland which is also of great importance in resistance to allergy.

Rapid Absorption. Sugar, like alcohol, is rapidly absorbed, and floods the system of the sensitive patient, predisposing him to severe reactions and addiction.

Degenerative Conditions. An overwhelming body of scientific evidence now shows that sugar is deleterious to general health, being implicated as a causative agent of importance in diabetes, dental caries, and other degenerative conditions such as hardening of the arteries and its complications (heart attack, stroke, and gangrene).

Depletes Nutrients. Sugar depletes the body of specific nutrients including the B vitamins and minerals, especially magnesium and chromium. You can change your own favorite recipes to eliminate sugar, using this formula:

Substitution of Honey

1. 1 cup honey contains ¼ cup liquid.
2. Deduct ¼ cup liquid from recipe when using honey in place of sugar.
3. Use ½ cup honey in place of 1 cup sugar.

* Dr. Warren Levin of Brooklyn, New York, was the physician who first demonstrated to us the dangers of sugars. It was his advice and counseling that led us to delete from our diet all crystallized sugar and to keep other sweeteners, such as honey, to a minimum. We are especially grateful to Dr. Levin for preparing this introduction.

Contents

BEVERAGES

Apple Beverage
(*milk free*)

1 pound apples, pared and cut in
small pieces
1 cup apple juice

½ cup nuts
lemon juice

Put ingredients in blender at high speed.

Banana Shake
(*milk free*)

2 tablespoons soya milk
1 pint water
1 large banana

1–2 pinches powdered vanilla
bean

Put ingredients in blender at high speed.

Banana Shake 2

1 part goat's milk
2 parts frozen banana

Pinch of nutmeg, cinnamon, or
drop of vanilla

Let bananas thaw just enough to cut up. Put ingredients in blender at medium speed. When bananas have formed a puree, blend at high speed. (Persons on a rotary diet can make a full meal using shake made with 4–6 bananas.)

Comfrey Drink
(*milk free, egg free, wheat free*)

15 almonds
5 teaspoons sunflower seeds
(soak overnight in water)
16 ounces juice

4 pitted dates
4 large handfuls of comfrey and
other greens (see below)

Fill the liquefier above the blades with unsweetened juice (approximately 8 ounces). Add softened nuts, seeds, and dates to the juice and liquefy. Pour this mixture into a pitcher. Next, take four large handfuls of green leaves, such as alfalfa, parsley, mint, spinach, beet greens, watercress and, most important, *comfrey*. Liquefy the greens in 8 ounces unsweetened juice. Combine the two mixtures, making sure the combination is not too thick. The mixture may be put through a coarse sieve or strainer.

Fruit Shake

(milk free, egg free)

2 tablespoons soya milk powder   4 dates, figs, prunes, or ¼ cup
1 pint water   raisins

Blend first at low speed, then at high speed.

Goat's Milk Shake

See Banana Shake 2

Instant Hot Drink

½ cup lemon juice   ½ cup honey

Mix together and freeze in half-pint jar. Mixture stays slushy rather than becoming solid. For a quick, hot drink, add 1 or 2 teaspoons to a cup of hot water. Return jar to freezer.

Juice Combinations

Try these delicious combinations:

Orange juice, bananas, papaya   —Liquefy in blender
Orange juice, cashew nuts   —Liquefy
Pineapple juice, carrots, celery   —Liquefy
Melon, coconut, bananas   —Liquefy
Apricot juice, almonds, rosehips
    powder, bananas   —Liquefy
Invent your own.

Marjoram Milk

For a soothing cup late at night, a sprig of sweet marjoram in a cup of warm milk.

Milk Shake

Chill dried skim milk in freezer compartment, then whip.

Variation:

Add cinnamon or nutmeg and/or a herb for flavoring.

Sesame Cream
(milk free)

Blend:

1 cup sesame seeds	dash powdered vanilla beans
1 cup warm water (blend smooth)	

Variation:

Sweeten with banana, dates, or figs.

BISCUITS, CRACKERS, AND MUFFINS

Corn Muffins
(wheat free, milk free)

2 egg yolks	2 heaping tablespoons cornmeal
1 tablespoon corn oil	1½ cups corn flour
1 cup sunflower seed milk	2 stiffly beaten egg whites

Preheat oven to 425° F. Beat the egg yolks and oil together, add the milk and cornmeal; then beat in the corn flour. Fold in the beaten egg whites last. Pour batter in oiled muffin tins and bake about 20 minutes.

Potato or Tapioca Flour Muffins

4 eggs	1 tablespoon honey
¼ teaspoon salt	½ cup potato or tapioca starch
4 tablespoons ice water	1 teaspoon baking powder

Preheat oven to 350° F. Separate eggs. Beat yolks and add salt and honey. Add water, sifted flour, and baking powder. Fold in stiffly beaten whites. Bake 15–20 minutes.

Pumpkin Seed Crackers
(wheat free, milk free, egg free)

3 cups pumpkin seed (before grinding)

Grind seed, then add:

1 cup ground sesame seeds	3 tablespoons oil
¾ teaspoon salt	

Preheat oven to 250° F. Add boiling water to make stiff dough. Oil cookie sheet and roll thin as possible on sheet. (Keep roller wet with water). Bake at 250° F. for 10 minutes, then at 350° F. for 15 minutes.

Variation:

The same recipe can be made with corn meal, corn flour, or sunflower seed in place of pumpkin seed.

Rice Wafers
(wheat free, egg free, milk free)

½ cup rice (gritty)
½ cup rice polish
½ teaspoon baking powder
½ teaspoon salt

1 tablespoon tapioca starch
½ cup almonds, ground
½ cup maple syrup or honey
⅜ cup oil

Preheat oven to 425° F. Mix ingredients. Pat batter into 9″ × 9″ oiled pan. Bake 10–20 minutes.

Soybean Muffins
(wheat free, milk free)

1⅔ cups soy flour
3½ teaspoons baking powder
½ teaspoon salt
2 eggs beaten

⅓ cup oil
⅓ cup honey
1⅓ cups water

Preheat oven to 350° F. Mix and bake for 20 minutes.

Sunflower Seed Wafer
(wheat free, milk free, egg free)

Put sunflower seed in blender and blend quite fine. Mix with water moist enough to handle. Make patties about ¼″ thick.

Preheat oven to 275° F. Bake on ungreased sheet at moderate temperature until brown. Turn and brown other side.

BREAD

Hints on Bread Making

Always have kitchen warm when making bread. Avoid drafts. The oven is an excellent place for bread to rise. Turn oven on and set at *warm* for five minutes before turning off again. Water must be lukewarm before adding yeast. To "punch down" simply beat bread with your fist. This helps the fermentation or yeast growth by moving the yeast cells to a new food supply, so that they can grow and multiply. Except for the flour used on hands and beneath bread while kneading, do not add flour after fermentation has begun.

Banana Nut Bread
(wheat free, milk free)

2 eggs
2 tablespoons water
1½ cups mashed banana
1½ cups arrowroot starch

½ teaspoon salt
1 teaspoon soda
¾ cup chopped pecans

Preheat oven to 350° F. Beat eggs. Combine water and banana; add to eggs alternately with dry ingredients. Mix thoroughly. Add nut meats. Bake in a lightly oiled 1-pound pan about ¾ hour.

Variations:

Substitute one cup stewed apricots (put through a food ricer or strainer) for the bananas.

Substitute 1½ cups applesauce for bananas plus ¼ teaspoon cloves and ½ teaspoon cinnamon.

Banana Oat Bread
(wheat free, milk free, egg free)

2 cups oat flour
1 teaspoon soda
¼ teaspoon salt
1 egg (¼ cup water may be
    substituted)

1 mashed banana
⅓ cup safflower oil
½ cup honey
½ cup chopped nuts or raisins

Preheat oven to 375° F. Mix all ingredients and add additional water if needed for right consistency. Bake in loaf pan about 25–30 minutes.

Coconut Bread
(wheat free, milk free,)

1 cup water (milk if allowed) or
    milk substitute
1½ cup soy bean flour
½ cup coconut

3 teaspoons baking powder
1 egg well beaten
2 tablespoons oil
½ teaspoon salt

Preheat oven to 350° F. Combine all ingredients. Bake in greased, floured loaf pan approximately 30 minutes.

Corn Bread
(wheat free, milk free, egg free)

1 cup cornmeal
¼ cup oil
½ cup water

1 teaspoon salt
1 teaspoon baking powder

Preheat oven to 450° F. Mix all ingredients. Pour batter into oiled 9″ × 9″ pan. Bake 10–15 minutes.

Date Bread
(wheat free, egg free, milk free)

1 cup chopped dates
1½ cups warm water
2 teaspoons baking soda
1 cup shortening or oil
⅓ cup honey

2 teaspoons baking powder
1 cup arrowroot, potato, or
   sesame flour
1 teaspoon sea salt

Preheat oven to 350° F. Let dates soak until water cools, then add baking soda. Add shortening or oil, honey, baking powder, flour, and salt. Bake 45 minutes in greased loaf pan.

Oatmeal Sheet Bread
(wheat free, egg free, milk free)

1 cup oat flour
1 tablespoon tapioca starch
¾ teaspoon salt

2 teaspoons baking powder
3 tablespoons oil
½ cup water

Preheat oven to 475° F. Mix all ingredients. Pat batter into 9″ × 9″ oiled pan. Bake 10–15 minutes.

Oatmeal Sheet Bread with Nuts
(wheat free, egg free, milk free)

1 cup oat flour
1 tablespoon tapioca starch
1 teaspoon salt
⅔ cup water

2 teaspoons baking powder
2 tablespoons oil
⅓ cup nuts (almonds good)

Preheat oven to 475° F. Mix ingredients. Pat batter into oiled 9″ × 9″ pan. Bake 10–20 minutes.

Peanut Bread
(milk free, wheat free)

1 cup peanut flour
½ teaspoon salt
3 teaspoons baking powder
1 tablespoon melted whole fat or
   2 teaspoons oil

1 egg
¾ cup water
2 tablespoons honey

Preheat oven to 350° F. Sift flour before measuring. Mix dry ingredients. Chop in fat. Beat egg, add water and honey, and blend with dry ingredients. Bake in 4″ × 7″ × 2″ pan 40 minutes.

Rice Sheet Bread
(milk free, wheat free, egg free)

1 cup rice flour	2 teaspoons baking powder
1 tablespoon tapioca starch	¾ cup water
1¼ teaspoons salt	2 tablespoons oil

Preheat oven to 425° F. Mix ingredients. Oil pan 9″ × 9″. Pat batter into pan. Bake 20–30 minutes.

Rye Baking Powder Bread
(milk free, wheat free, egg free)

1½ cups plus 2 tablespoons whole rye flour	4 teaspoons whole melted fat or 3½ teaspoons oil
¼ teaspoon salt	½ cup water
5 teaspoons baking powder	

Preheat oven to 375° F. Sift flour before measuring. Mix dry ingredients. Chop in fat and add water, beating with long stroke. Bake in 4″ × 9″ × 2″ pan 20 minutes.

Variation:

If allowed, 2 eggs may be added, reducing flour to 1¼ cups.

Sesame Bread
(milk free, wheat free)

¾ cup sesame seed meal	½ teaspoon salt
¾ cup arrowroot starch	1 egg, well beaten
2 teaspoons baking powder	2 tablespoons sesame oil
½ cup water, milk, or equivalent	

Preheat oven to 375° F. Mix thoroughly. Place in greased, starch-floured 4″ × 7″ × 2″ pan. Bake 30 minutes.

Soy Loaf Bread
(wheat free, milk free, egg free)

1 cup arrowroot starch	2 tablespoons honey
1 tablespoon baking powder	3 tablespoons soy oil
2 cups soy flour	2 cups water
1 teaspoon salt	

Preheat oven to 375° F. Mix dry ingredients. Blend honey, oil, and water and stir into dry ingredients. Bake in 2 small pans, 3″ × 6″, 35 minutes.

Spoon Bread
(wheat free)

3 cups milk
1 cup cornmeal
1½ teaspoons salt

2 tablespoons butter
4 egg yolks, beaten
4 egg whites

Preheat oven to 400° F. Combine milk, cornmeal, and salt. Cook over low heat, stirring constantly until thickened. Add fat. Cool mixture. Stir in egg yolks. Beat egg whites until stiff, but not dry. Fold into cornmeal mixture. Pour into greased 1½ quart casserole. Bake 35–40 minutes. Makes 6 servings.

Whole Wheat Sesame Bread
(milk free, egg free)

3¾ cups or more hot water
7 tablespoons honey
½ cup ground sesame seed
1 package Red Star yeast
¼ cup warm water

9 cups whole wheat flour
   (approximately)
1 tablespoon salt
¼ cup sesame seed oil

Preheat oven to 350° F. Combine hot water, oil, honey, and sesame seed. Cool to lukewarm. Add yeast to ¼ cup *warm* water. Mix well. Add to other liquids only after they have been cooled to lukewarm. Blend 5 cups of the flour with salt and the liquids. Let stand in warm place for at least two hours. Blend in additional flour until dough is stiff. Knead for approximately 6 minutes. Put dough back in bowl, oil top, cover, and let rise for one hour. Punch down. Knead again. Divide into two loaves and place in oiled loaf pans. Let rise again until double in bulk. Bake 50 minutes to an hour.

CAKES

Carob Angel Food Cake
(wheat free, milk free)

1 cup of carob powder

12 egg whites

Preheat oven to 300° F. Add carob powder to egg whites and beat until very light. Bake from 20–30 minutes.

Carob Cake
(wheat free, milk free)

1 cup carob powder
12 eggs

12 egg whites (if large, 8 eggs
and 8 egg whites should do)

Preheat oven to 300° F. Add carob powder to eggs and egg whites and whip until light. Bake, in an ungreased cake pan, a little longer than the carob angel food cake or until done. Invert in pan on rack to cool.

Carrot Cake
(milk free, wheat free)

1 cup grated raw carrots
¾ cup grated or shredded
   coconut
1 cup honey
½" vanilla bean, powdered

1 cup grated raw cashew nuts
   (¼ lb)
6 eggs
½ teaspoon salt
¾ teaspoon cream of tartar

Preheat oven to 450° F. Combine carrots, coconut, and honey. Add vanilla to the mixture and blend. Let stand for 1 hour so coconut will absorb moisture of carrots. Separate eggs. Add salt to egg yolks, beat to a creamy consistency. Fold egg yolks into the carrot and coconut mixture. Add grated nuts and blend. Beat egg whites until stiff and sprinkle cream of tartar over them as you continue beating. (This should be done with a wire beater to incorporate lots of air.) When egg whites are dry, fold into the combined ingredients, pour into an angel food cake pan with a loose bottom or if another pan is used, better have the removable bottom. Do not grease. Bake at 450° F. for 25 minutes, then at 350° F. for 20–25 minutes more, or until cake shows signs of leaving the sides of the pan. Remove from oven and turn upside down until cool. Use thin knife to cut cake from bottom and side of pan. This cake does not need icing as it is rich and dainty.

Holly Berry Fruit Cake
(milk free, wheat free, egg free)

Prepare at least a week before Christmas. Grind the following ingredients through food chopper and place in large mixing bowl:

1 cup pitted dates
1 cup stemmed figs
1 cup raisins
1 cup pitted prunes

1 cup sunflower seeds
1 cup raw coconut chunks
   (optional)

Add the following ingredients and blend together:

4 egg yolks
1 cup plumped raisins
1 cup red frozen cherries
     (thawed)

1 cup raw honey (add more later
     if needed)
1 cup whole nut meats
½ cup pignolias

Now add enough raw peanut flour to make a very stiff raw dough. Pack in oiled bread tins, wrap in towels, and put in cold place to ripen. Garnish before serving by cutting holly leaves out of salad greens and cutting small berries out of thawed red cherries.

Peach Cobbler
(wheat free, milk free, egg free)

4 cups sliced peaches (or apples)
2 tablespoons tapioca

½ cup honey
½ teaspoon salt

Mix and add:
1 cup soy flour
½ teaspoon salt
6 tablespoons soy oil

1 teaspoon baking powder
¼ cup honey
⅓ cup water

Bake in preheated oven at 400° F. for 25–30 minutes.

Protein Cake
(wheat free, milk free)

7 eggs, separated
⅓ cup honey
1 teaspoon vanilla

pinch salt
½ pound nuts, ground fine

Preheat oven to 325° F. Beat egg whites until stiff, blend honey, vanilla, and salt with egg yolks. Add nuts and mix well. Fold into whites. Place in ungreased angel food cake pan and bake 1 hour. Invert and when cool, remove from the pan.

Soy Honey Cake
(wheat free, milk free, egg free)

Sift together:
⅔ cup soy flour
3 teaspoons baking powder
½ teaspoon sea salt

⅓ cup potato (arrowroot or
     tapioca) flour

Add 3 tablespoons soy oil and ¾ cup honey alternately with ½ cup water. Bake in round cake pan in preheated oven at 375° F. for 30 minutes.

CANDIES AND SNACKS

Almond Sweets

1 cup sesame seeds	½ cup almonds

Put through food chopper, form into balls, and roll in coconut.

Apricot Marbles

1 cup sun-dried apricots	½ pound coconut
½ cup nut meats	4 tablespoons lemon juice

Put apricots, nuts, and coconut through food chopper. Add lemon juice. Shape into balls; roll in chopped nuts.

Coconut Molasses Chews

½ cup honey	½ cup molasses
1 tablespoon vinegar, lime, or lemon juice	2 tablespoons butter
	2¼ cups moist coconut

Stir and cook all ingredients except coconut over quick heat until they boil. Cover with lid for 3 minutes. Continue cooking, stirring occasionally until the syrup reaches the firm-ball stage, 248° F. Remove from heat. Work in coconut with 2 forks. When slightly cooled, dip fingers into ice water and shape into balls. Note: Maple syrup may be used in place of honey. If so, do not cook quite so long.

Date Delight

1 cup chopped pitted dates	1 cup chopped nuts
½ cup maple syrup	2 egg yolks
2 heaping teaspoons wheat germ flour (make your own by whizzing ½ cup wheat germ in blender)	2 egg whites

Preheat oven to 300° F. Cream these ingredients together while egg whites are being beaten stiff in electric mixer. Fold in beaten whites and pour batter in 9″ × 9″ cake pan. Bake 30 minutes, or until toothpick comes out clean.

Date Patties

1 cup dates	1 cup pecans

Put through food chopper, form into balls and roll in coconut or ground nuts.

Cheese Stuffed Dates

Remove pits from dates and stuff with pieces of cheese. Roll in freshly grated coconut.

Honey Taffy

2 cups honey
1 tablespoon butter   pinch sea salt

Gently simmer the honey until it reaches the hard-ball stage, remove from fire, add salt and butter, and pour in a buttered pan. Let cool, then pull.

NUTS

Note: One pound of nuts in the shell will yield about ½ pound of nut meats. To shell hard-shell nuts more easily (filberts, walnuts, pecans, butternuts): pour boiling water over the nuts and let stand 15 minutes. Drain.

Hints on Blanching Nuts

To blanch *brazil nuts:* cover with boiling water, bring back to a boil and boil 3 minutes. Drain and cool. To blanch *almonds and pistachios:* remove shell and cover with boiling water. Let stand 2 minutes. Drain and put into cold water. Rub off skin with the fingers and dry nuts with soft, clean cloth. To blanch *chestnuts:* cut a ½" crisscross gash on the flat side with a sharp paring knife. Cover the nuts with water and bring slowly to the boiling point. Take out nuts, one by one, and remove the shell and inner skin with a sharp, pointed knife. To blanch *filberts:* shell nuts. Cover with boiling water. Let stand 6 minutes. Drain. Remove skins with sharp knife.

Raisin and Nut Balls
(*milk free, wheat free, egg free*)

2 parts seeded raisins   1 part filberts

Put through food chopper, form into balls and roll in sesame seed, coconut, or nut meal.

Nut and Seed Balls
(egg free)

1 cup squash seed meal
½ cup sesame seeds
2 tablespoons carob
dash of pure vanilla

1 cup sunflower seed meal
½ cup chopped nuts
2 tablespoons honey
2 tablespoons cream

Mix all ingredients and cream together well. Form into balls. Roll in coconut.

Snow Balls

4 cups dried fruit

1½ cups blanched coconut or
    almonds or other nuts

Toss together fruit and ½ cup almonds or coconut. Prepare meat grinder by pouring hot water through to prevent sticking. Force mixture through grinder. With moistened hands shape into ¾″ balls. If using nuts, finely chop remaining cup. If using coconut, finely grate remaining cup or use shredded coconut. Roll balls in nuts or coconut to coat. Store in covered jar. Makes about 6 dozen.

Variation:

For flavor add rind of ½ orange (orange part only) stripped with vegetable peeler.

Sesame Seed Candy

2 cups sesame seed
½ cup oil
2 tablespoons honey

½ teaspoon vanilla
1 tablespoon peanut butter
1 tablespoon carob powder

Put in blender sesame seeds and oil. Start blender with cover on and run it for one minute. Take the cover off and help push seeds down and under. Add honey and vanilla; blend until smooth. Divide into three bowls. Add peanut butter to one, carob to another, leave one plain. Shape.

St. Nick Candies

½ cup nuts
1 cup pitted dates
1 cup raisins

½ cup sunflower seeds
1 cup figs
honey, as needed

Put all ingredients through the food chopper; add enough honey to make mixture which will pack in a 9″ × 9″ square Pyrex baking dish. Cut in squares, place a large, red, dried sweet cherry in center of each one. Dip sides and bottom in sesame seeds.

Sunflower Seed Candy

2 cups sunflower seeds
1 heaping tablespoon honey
1 cup of ground seeds

1 heaping tablespoon peanut
    butter
dash of vanilla

Put in blender sunflower seeds and grind to a fine meal. Start with cover on, then remove cover and push seeds down with spatula. Always do this carefully, keeping far away from the knife. Add honey to 1 cup of the ground seeds, peanut butter and dash of vanilla to the other cup. Stir well into dough; form into balls or desired shapes and roll in coating mixtures.

COOKIES

Almond Cookies
(wheat free, milk free, egg free)

Grind 3 cups almonds (measure
    before grinding)
½ teaspoon cinnamon
1 tablespoon lemon juice plus
    grated rind

3 tablespoons honey
½ teaspoon salt
1½ tablespoons oil

Preheat oven to 250° F. Mix all ingredients. Add boiling water gradually to make stiff dough. Oil cookie sheets. Roll out on sheets as thinly as possible. (Keep roller wet with water.) Cut in squares. Bake about 25 minutes. Should be chewy rather than hard.

Carob Artichoke Cookies
(wheat free, milk free, egg free)

2 cups Jerusalem artichoke flour
½ cup toasted carob flour
½ teaspoon salt
½ cup oil
1 teaspoon baking powder

¾ cup maple syrup
¼ teaspoon ginger powder
2–4 tablespoons water to make
    dough

Preheat oven to 350° F. Combine ingredients. Roll dough. Cut square cookies with knife or round ones with rim of small glass. Bake until done.

Carob Cookies
(milk free, wheat free)

3 egg whites   ½ cup carob powder

Preheat oven to 300° F. Beat egg whites until very stiff, then fold in carob powder with spatula. Drop on a greased cookie sheet and bake 15 minutes. You may add a few nuts to each cookie before baking if you wish. Honey may be added, if desired, but cookies are actually sweet enough with just the carob powder.

Raw Coconut Cookies
(wheat free, milk free, egg free)

1 cup grated or ground coconut

Use enough honey to hold the coconut together. Form into small cookies, press a whole nut meat in each center and keep in refrigerator until ready to serve.

Coconut Molasses Chews
(wheat free, egg free)

½ cup honey   2½ cups moist coconut
1 tablespoon vinegar, lime or   ½ cup molasses
    lemon juice   2 tablespoons butter

Stir and cook these ingredients over high heat until they boil. Cover them with lid for 3 minutes. Continue cooking, stirring occasionally until the syrup reaches the firm-ball stage, 248° F. Remove from heat. Work in coconut with 2 forks. When slightly cooled, dip fingers into ice water and shape into balls. Note: Maple syrup may be used in place of honey. If so, do not cook quite so long.

Date Coconut Cookies
(wheat free, milk free, egg free)

1 cup dates, chopped   ¼ teaspoon salt
1 cup shredded coconut   spring water as needed
½ teaspoon soda   1 teaspoon oil
⅓ cup tapioca starch or arrowroot

Preheat oven to 375° F. Cover dates with water, bring to boil, and cool. Mix together all dry ingredients and add dates, water, and oil. Drop on greased cookie sheets. Bake until brown (10–12 minutes).

Rice Cookies
(milk free, wheat free, egg free)

¼ cup water	½ cup rice flour
¼ cup raisins	⅛ cup oil
¼ cup filberts	½ teaspoon baking powder
½ teaspoon salt	

Preheat oven to 400° F. Mix ingredients. Form batter into balls and flatten on oiled cookie sheet. Bake 5–7 minutes.

Rice Almond Cookies
(wheat free, egg free, milk free)

⅔ cup sweet (glutenous) rice— grind to flour	⅛ teaspoon ground vanilla bean
⅓ cup almonds (before grinding)	⅛ teaspoon sea salt
finely grated orange peel, to taste (approximately ½ teaspoon)	1 teaspoon oil
	½ cup water

Preheat oven to 300° F. Mix well, adding water last. Drop from teaspoon and flatten with fingertips. Bake approximately 30 minutes.

Soy Cookies
(wheat free)

1 cup soy flour	2 teaspoons baking powder
1 cup arrowroot flour (or tapioca)	¾ cup honey
4 tablespoons butter (or oil)	add 1 cup nuts or seeds for body
½ teaspoon salt	

Preheat oven to 325° F. Roll out ¼" thick. Cut cookies 1¼" to 1½" across. Bake 15–17 minutes.

DAIRY FOODS

Blended Butter

1 pound butter	1 cup safflower (or other oil)
1 pinch salt	

Soften butter to room temperature. Using electric mixer, blend in salt. Gradually blend in oil. When refrigerated, it will spread easily. Per unit volume, lower in saturated fats. Less expensive. Taste is good.

Country Cottage Cheese

Heat sour milk until the whey (clear liquid) comes to the top. Do not boil! Pour off the whey and put the curd into a cheesecloth bag. Drain for 6 hours. Put it into a bowl and chop to desired coarseness. Salt to taste. Add cream if you wish, or work it to the texture of soft putty (paste) adding a little cream and butter as needed. Mold with hands into pats or balls. Keep in a cool place. Best when fresh.

Sour Cream
(low fat)

Make cottage cheese (above). Add as little milk as necessary for it to whip in blender. If onion or herbs are to be added, do this before using blender.

Yogurt

2 cups fresh milk

2 heaping tablespoons sour cream

Heat milk slowly until lukewarm (just warm when a few drops are spilled on wrist). Remove from heat. Pour into wide-mouth jar. Add sour cream or milk. Stir briskly. Cover. Set aside in warm place. When thickened, chill several hours or overnight. Serve with fruit or vegetables. You may sweeten and flavor with vanilla. Dry commercial yogurt cultures can be purchased. Starters taken from such a batch are effective only for one month. For economy, freeze this batch as individual ice cubes. Use one cube each month for your new starter.

DESSERTS

Apples Stuffed with Sweet Potatoes

6 medium apples
1 teaspoon cinnamon
3 tablespoons honey
1 tablespoon butter

2 cups mashed cooked sweet potato
½ teaspoon sea salt

Cut apples in half and remove core. Place on baking pan and sprinkle with cinnamon and honey. Bake slowly until tender. Prepare sweet potato filling by adding other ingredients and mixing well. Fill cooked apples with potato. Serve hot.

Glazed Apples

Preheat oven to 350° F. Pare and core small tart apples. Place in greased baking pan or casserole and sprinkle with honey. Add small amount of water. Bake uncovered for about ½ hour or until tender. Baste syrup over apples 2 or 3 times during cooking for an attractive glaze. Fill centers with raisins and serve.

Carob Pudding
(wheat free, egg free)

3¼ cups water, milk, or milk
    substitute
3 tablespoons potato starch
3 tablespoons carob (toasted
    flour)

3 tablespoons butter (if allowed)
dash of salt
¾ cup maple syrup

Mix to thicken. Stir while cooking.

Dried Fruits

Steam: Put a raised rack or trivet (to allow circulation of steam) in pot with tight lid. The rack can be raised above water level with 2 or 3 suitable metal objects. Add enough water (spring or distilled) so that the pot will not boil dry. Place dried fruit in one layer on rack. Cover tightly and steam 10–15 minutes or more if not yet tender. Can be eaten as is or stuffed with other fruit, nuts, cheese, meat, and rolled in dried coconut, grated nuts, or ground seed, or wrap in cookie dough or pie crust and bake, or chop and use in any way.

Variation:

Instead of steaming, soak the dried fruit in spring water or juice for 24 to 48 hours. This preserves all vitamins, minerals and enzymes.
    Combine with other ingredients as indicated above.

Gelatin Dessert

One package gelatin plus 2 cups any fruit juice and honey to taste. Soften gelatin in 1 cup of above liquid and dissolve by heating. Then add remaining liquid. Add fruit and nuts if desired. Mold and chill.

Honey-Mint Sauce for Puddings
(wheat free, milk free)

1 cup light honey
2 egg whites

dash of salt
1 teaspoon minced curly mint

Heat the honey, beat egg whites and salt. Then stir in honey in a fine stream, continuing to beat until all honey is added. Garnish with mint leaves.

Banana Ice Cream
(wheat free, egg free)

2 bananas
1½ cups milk
Lemon or orange juice to taste

3 tablespoons honey
2 tablespoons safflower oil

Mix in blender or mash bananas and mix together with electric beater. Freeze, whip again, and refreeze.

Maple Ice Cream
(sugar free, milk free)

In a mixing bowl put the following:

1 scant cup maple syrup
4 egg yolks

⅛ teaspoon powdered vanilla
bean
1 cup ground nut meats

Beat until mixture is very creamy. Fold in 4 stiffly beaten egg whites, pour into refrigerator tray, and freeze at lowest point of dial. Beat mixture with spoon 3 times during freezing.

Variation:
Use sunflower seeds in place of nuts. Use honey in place of the maple syrup. Leave the nuts whole.

Maple Velvet Cream

1 tablespoon plain gelatin
2 eggs, separated
½ cup cold water

⅛ teaspoon salt
1½ cups hot maple syrup
1 cup whipping cream

In the top of a double boiler (on kitchen counter), soak the gelatin in the cold water for 5 minutes. Stir in egg yolks and salt. Then stir in hot maple syrup and place over boiling water and stir until it thickens slightly. Cover and cook 10 minutes stirring once or twice. Cool and chill over cold water. Stir frequently until it begins to set. Fold in stiffly beaten egg whites and whipped cream. Turn into stemware or cut glass bowl. Refrigerate until serving time.

Molasses Butter
(milk free, egg free)

2 cups cooked apples

1 cup molasses (maple syrup, honey)

Cook well, stirring constantly, until thick and buttery. Good with sweet potatoes or pumpkin, as well as a spread.

Popsicles

Put fruits through the blender and strainer or the clear juicer and freeze these juices into popsicles for the children.

Rhubarb Custard
(sugar free, milk free)

1 egg beaten
¼ cup water
2 tablespoons maple syrup or raisins (optional)
nutmeg (optional)

1 tablespoon allowed starch
pinch of salt
thin slices rhubarb (floats on top)
½ stalk

Preheat oven to 300° F. Mix well, pour into baking dish, set dish in pan of water and bake for 30 minutes to set egg (uncovered).

Sherbet
(milk free)

1 cup fruit juice or mashed organic berries
2 egg whites beaten stiff (may be omitted if allergic to eggs)

2 cups water
⅔ cup honey

Boil water and honey for 5 minutes. Cool and add fruit juice and put in freezing tray. When firm, remove and mix with stiffly beaten egg whites, beating mixture with electric mixer until light and frothy.

Vegetable Pudding
(milk free, egg free)

½ cup oil, butter or fat
4 cups grated or ground starchy,

raw vegetable (carrot and potato a good combination)

Add and mix in order:
½ cup honey
2 teaspoons baking powder
1 teaspoon soda

1 teaspoon salt
1 teaspoon cinnamon
1 cup raisins (or any dried fruit)

Preheat oven to 350° F. Grease pan. Oven steam for 1 hour or bake for ¾ hour.

DRESSINGS, FLAVORINGS, MAYONNAISES AND SPREADS

Avocado Salad Dressing

1 ripe avocado
½ lemon minus peel

juice of ½ orange

Cube avocado into blender with orange juice. Pit lemon and cut into blender. Blend at medium speed. Delicious on celery, fish, lobster. Celery or carrot juice may be substituted for citrus juice.

Butter Sauce

To ¼ cup butter (or tolerated vegetable oil) heated, add *one* of the following and cook, stirring constantly:

2 tablespoons grated cheese
1 tablespoon grated celery
Few grains grated garlic
1 tablespoon lemon juice
1 teaspoon grated lemon rind

2 tablespoons grated onion
2 tablespoons vinegar
¼ teaspoon tolerated herbs
¼ cup orange juice

Add 2 tablespoons of any of above to hot, cooked vegetables, meat, fish, or poultry.

Chives

Chives, "the garlic without regret," rosemary, and parsley minced in melted butter can be painted on a roast with a small brush kept for that purpose.

Easy Mayonnaise Dip

In blender:
1 egg or 2 egg yolks
½ cup cider vinegar
½ cup honey

2 teaspoons kelp or sea salt
vegetable oil

For best results, all ingredients should be at room temperature. Start blender and remove cover. While blender is running, pour vegetable oil in steady stream down the middle until the ingredients begin to thicken and the oil lies on top. Blend until thick and heavy. Add color with bits of red and green pepper, parsley, celery, pickles. Put this in a bowl in center of platter, or, for a novelty, hollow out a pepper or other vegetable and fill that with the dip.

French Dressing

3 parts oil

1 part lemon juice or vinegar
(more if desired)

Add lemon juice slowly to oil.

Italian Dressing

1 clove garlic
1 teaspoon honey
1 teaspoon mustard

1 tablespoon lemon juice
2 tablespoons oil
chopped mint

Pound garlic until smooth. Add honey and mustard. Stir until smooth, then add lemon juice drop by drop and beat well. Add the oil gradually and then a sprinkling of chopped mint.

Mayonnaise

2 egg yolks
1 cup oil

1 teaspoon salt
lemon juice or cider vinegar

For best results, all ingredients should be at room temperature. Beat salt into unbeaten egg yolks. Add oil very slowly, drop by drop at first, until the dressing becomes thick and shiny. (If it curdles, add another yolk, beating this in slowly also.) After ½ cup oil has been used, add 1 tablespoon lemon juice or vinegar. Then continue to add the oil teaspoon by teaspoon.

Mayonnaise 2
(egg free)

¼ cup vinegar or lemon juice
1 teaspoon salt
¼–1 cup mashed potato (hot or
    cold, hot preferred)

¾ cup oil
1 teaspoon honey
pinch of flavored herbs (optional)

Blend all ingredients in blender or with mixer. Refrigerate. It will thicken as it cools.

Blender Mayonnaise

1 egg
¾ teaspoon salt
½ teaspoon dry mustard

2 tablespoons vinegar
1 cup oil

Put egg, seasonings, vinegar and ¼ cup of oil into blender and process at blend speed (high speed in a 3–speed blender). Immediately remove top and gradually pour in remaining oil in a steady stream. Turn off. If oil remains, stir with spoon and blend a few seconds more. Repeat until oil disappears.

If the mayonnaise does not thicken, pour the batter back into the measuring cup leaving ¼ cup in the blender, add an egg and process at blend speed, removing top and gradually pouring in the remaining batter in a steady stream.

Mint Sauce

¼ cup chopped fresh mint
1 tablespoon honey

½ cup wine vinegar
pinch salt

Combine and allow to stand for 2 hours before using. For roasts, lamb, and rabbit.

Orange Flavoring

Blend dried peel of organic orange until it becomes a powder. Use this for flavoring in cakes, cookies, custards.

Uncooked Tomato Relish

4 quarts tomatoes
1½ cups chopped onion
¼ cup sweet red pepper
4 cups diced celery

2½ cups cider vinegar
¼ cup salt
2 tablespoons mustard seed

Chop tomatoes and onion fine and place in separate containers. Divide the salt between each and let stand for 3 hours. Combine and let stand overnight in the refrigerator. Add remaining ingredients and pack in sterile jars.

Peanut Butter

1 cup shelled peanuts

1 teaspoon peanut oil

Put peanuts and peanut oil in the blender. Blend, switching motor on and off to prevent overheating until you have the consistency you want. You can have anything from chunk style to smooth to sloppy. Keep in refrigerator. If you don't like unroasted peanuts, roast them for 20 minutes at 300° F. in their shells, and cool before using.

MEAT AND FOWL

Baked Chicken

Preheat oven to 350° F. Cut chicken in pieces, add fresh pineapple chunks, ginger root, stick cinnamon. Bake about 1 hour. As an alternative, bake chicken with organic cranberry juice and add quartered bananas the last half hour. Try this with guinea hen also.

Buffalo Stew

Slow-cook bones and pieces of buffalo. Add vegetables: Carrots, celery tops, parsnips, parsley, potatoes (optional). Season with: 1 tablespoon vinegar, specks of pepper and thyme, trace of rosemary (optional). Stew until broth is colored and thickened by vegetables (1 hour).

Roast Chicken

Rub salt and a pinch of herbs into a frozen fryer (3 pounds plus). Fasten legs together with bit of string. Cook in pressure cooker for 30 minutes or less. Remove with great care so it does not fall apart. Salt again and use herbs if desired. Broil until browned nicely, only a few minutes. Thicken broth in pressure cooker for gravy, using allowed starch.

Sesame Chicken or Guinea Hen

Preheat oven to 250° F. Dip chicken into beaten egg. Sprinkle generously with sesame seed meal (don't dip into the meal; when sesame meal is wet it doesn't cling to the chicken). Place in a baking dish (Pyrex cake dish is satisfactory) which has been greased with sesame seed oil. Bake 3–5 hours, depending on how crisp you like it. If you let it bake long enough, it becomes as crisp as fried chicken.

Country Pie

1–1½ pounds ground beef
1 tablespoon onion, chopped fine
1 teaspoon salt

2 tablespoons green pepper, (chopped fine)
4 or more cups Spanish rice (see Spanish rice recipe)

Preheat oven to 350° F. Combine beef, onion, pepper, and salt and press into pie tin as for a pie crust. Fill crust with Spanish rice. If desired, sprinkle over the top a little more salt and perhaps chopped chives. Cover with foil or an oven-proof lid of reasonable size. Bake 25 minutes. Uncover. Bake 10–15 minutes longer. Serve with grated cheese if desired.

Gnocci

½ cup melted suet or other
    animal fat
2 cups riced or mashed white
    potato

½ teaspoon baking powder
1 teaspoon salt
paprika
½ cup potato meal

Preheat oven to 400° F. Beat together well. Roll into cylinders 1½ inch in diameter. Chill. Cut into ¼ inch thick slices and indent with finger. Place in greased baking dish, edges overlapping. Cover with meat or tomato sauce. Bake 20 minutes. May be varied by using 1 egg in mix or by adding herbs. Serve with gravy, ham, chicken.

Goat Chops

Defat, salt, and cook until nearly done 4 or 5 goat chops.
Add:

1 tomato
2 tablespoons maple syrup
1 tablespoon chopped parsley
dash thyme

dash marjoram
speck of pepper
2 tablespoons white grape juice

Cook down, stirring constantly.

Lentil Soup with Meat

3 cups lentils
4 quarts water
1 cup chopped onions

2 bay leaves
3½ cups tomatoes
1 pound ground meat

Combine boiled water and lentils and simmer for 2 hours. Discard bay leaves. In a blender or food mill puree the mixture with 3½ cups tomatoes. Return pan to heat. Shape into ½" balls 1 pound ground meat. Add to the soup and simmer for 20 minutes. Salt to taste and serve.

Meat Balls

1½ pounds ground beef
¾ cup crumbed starch (cooked
    rice, dry cereal, raw oatmeal,
    nuts, grated raw or cooked
    potato, sweet potato,
    artichoke)

¼ cup onion, chopped fine
¼ cup green pepper, chopped
¼–½ teaspoon favorite herb
2 teaspoons salt
1 cup tomato juice (or equivalent,
    even water)

Shape into 16 balls. Brown in 1 or 2 tablespoons hot oil or fat. Turn heat low and allow to cook until done, approximately 25 to 30 minutes. You may add (after browning) tomato juice or equivalent and allow to simmer 20 to 25 minutes.

Meat Loaf

Preheat oven to 350° F. Combine ingredients for meat balls in preceding recipe. Use standard-size bread pan, greased. Bake 1 hour. Let stand 5 minutes or so for easier slicing. May use greased muffin pan and bake for approximately 20 minutes.

Basic Meat Loaf

1½ pounds ground meat
¼ to ½ cup starch

1½ teaspoon salt
½ to 1 cup liquid

Preheat oven to 325° F. Mix well, form into loaf. Bake 1½ hours.

For ground meat use: ground beef, buffalo, goat, lamb, pork.

For starch use: potato meal, riced cooked potato, raw grated potato, grated carrots, tapioca, arrowroot.

For liquid use: meat juice/or gravy, tomato juice, milk or milk substitute.

Season with: ⅛ teaspoon marjoram and ⅛ teaspoon thyme or ¼ teaspoon rosemary and ¼ teaspoon savory or 1 tablespoon lemon juice and grated lemon rind or 1 cup chopped celery or 1 cup chopped onion. Chopped cooked liver may be mixed with the ground meat.

Meat Sauce

2 quarts tomato juice or 1 quart whole tomatoes to 1 pound ground meat (in large quantities, put more meat in proportion to juice)

Oregano (½ teaspoon per pound of meat up to 1½ teaspoons)
Add bits of green pepper to taste

Flake meat. Put all ingredients together and cook on medium heat, then simmer about 3½–4 hours. Freeze if desired.

Meat Balls

1 pound ground meat
½ cup rice, raw
2–4 teaspoons finely chopped green pepper, if desired

1½ teaspoons salt
2 tablespoons onion, finely chopped

Mix and shape into 8—12 balls. Brown. Add 3½ cups tomatoes or equivalent. Simmer until done, 30—45 minutes, or cook in pressure cooker for 20 minutes.

Spanish Rice 1

Brown 1 to 1½ pounds ground meat

Add:

3½ cups tomatoes, raw or cooked	2 cups water (more if needed)
2 cups raw brown rice	2 tablespoons sea salt

Simmer until done. Stir occasionally. Cook rice, 45—75 minutes. Cooking time can be shortened by combining earlier the tomatoes, rice, water, and salt, thereby allowing the rice to soak.

Variation:

Add: 1 onion chopped, 1 green pepper chopped
    Italian flavor: ½ teaspoon oregano, ¼ teaspoon thyme, ¼ teaspoon cumin
    Spicy flavor: ½ teaspoon celery salt, ½ teaspoon basil

Spanish Rice 2

Brown buffalo meat and season with savory, rosemary, watercress, and salt. Cook: ½ cup rice in meat broth.

Add:

½ cup okra (previously cooked and drained)	1 cup tomato juice
	¼ cup celery tops, chopped

Simmer until juice disappears.

Variations:

Use as filling for baked, stuffed green peppers, tomatoes.
    Meat roll: using 1—1½ pounds ground meat and 1 teaspoon salt, roll the meat to make a rectangle 12″ × 15″. Spread the rice over this to a depth of no more than ½″. Then roll as for jelly roll. Bake as for Country Pie. Or you can make slices and place them cut side up in a dish and bake.
    Using seasoned ground beef, make thin patties 4″ across. Place a large spoonful Spanish rice in center of patty and turn up edges as for a tart. Place in covered frying pan and cook at 300° F. until the crust of rice is firm and browned.

Special Feature Recipe for Game Meat

Following is the recipe for "Unpalatable-Meat-Made-Palatable Sauce":

2 quarts tomato juice or 1 quart whole tomatoes to 1 pound ground meat. (In large quantities, put more meat in proportion to juice.)

oregano (½ teaspoon per pound of meat up to 1½ teaspoons)
green pepper to taste

Flake meat. Put all ingredients together and cook on medium heat, then simmer about 3½–4 hours. Freeze, if desired.

Squirrel

Four or five squirrels will serve five or six people. Dress, clean, and cut into serving pieces. Rub with lemon or vinegar and keep in refrigerator overnight. Wipe with a damp cloth, season, dust with flour or allowed starch, and fry as you would chicken, until brown, about 40 minutes. Cover with cream or rich chicken broth and roast in medium oven for 20 minutes.

Tame Tamale Pie

4 ounces meat (goat, rabbit, buffalo)
1 teaspoon salt
pinch of basil
pinch of oregano

pinch of thyme
dash chili or pepper
1 pint tomatoes
½ cup corn

Cook meat with seasonings. (Add onion if desired.) Add tomatoes and corn to meat mixture.

Turkey à la Gourmet

Preheat oven to 250° F. Remove fowl taste by salting (see Cooking Hints). Line the roasting pan generously with frozen green peppers. Use 1 cup green peppers for stuffing. Place in oven for 2 hours. Pour ¾ cup juice (grape or any berry juice) over turkey. Baste every 10 minutes for ½ hour. Leave in oven overnight at 250° F.

Jellied Veal Loaf

1 veal knuckle bone, sawed in half, or 2 tablespoons gelatin
1 pound diced veal
1 onion, sliced, if desired

bits of red (chopped tomato, red sweet pepper, if desired)
1 bay leaf, or ¼ to ½ teaspoon other herb, if desired

Combine and cover with water. Simmer 2 hours. Remove veal and bone. Chop meat into fine bits. Strain broth and cook down to make 1 cup. (If using gelatin, add to broth and stir until dissolved.) Oil loaf pan, sides and bottom. Add meat and slice with sharp knife. Veal bones and chicken bones will make a broth that jells. Other meats must have gelatin added. Veal has so mild a flavor that it needs added flavor from herbs or added vegetable juices (instead of water).

Preparing Hares and Rabbits

Cut off the legs at the first joints.

Slit the skin all along the belly and loosen it from the body. Pull it off the hind legs, then pull toward the head and off the front legs.

Slit the belly and draw out the entrails. Keep the liver and heart to use for making stock. Wash the animal well in cold water. Truss for roasting by skewering or tying legs close to the body or disjoint as follows:

Cut off the head, cut out the eyes and split the head in half lengthwise. Use it for stock.

Cut off the hind legs close to the body. The joints are quite easy to find.

Cut the body into three or four pieces through the backbone. The piece with the forelegs should be cut in half lengthwise.

Prepare as you would a chicken.

MISCELLANEOUS

Noodles, Tapioca
(wheat free, milk free)

Beat until light:
3 egg yolks   1 whole egg

Beat in:
3 tablespoons cold water   1 teaspoon salt

Stir in and work with hands:
2 cups tapioca starch

Divide flour into 3 parts. Roll out each piece as thinly as possible on lightly floured board. Place between 2 towels until dough is partially dried. Roll up dough as for jelly roll. Cut with sharp knife into strips of desired thickness. Shake out strips and allow to dry before using or storing.

Poi Soufflé

½ jar of poi
½ teaspoon salt
1 cup diced turkey
1 tablespoon chopped onion

2 egg yolks
1 tablespoon turkey gravy (grease removed)
2 egg whites

Preheat oven to 350° F. Put poi through a food mill or ricer. To it, add egg yolks, salt, onion, turkey gravy, and diced turkey. Use more gravy if necessary. Mix well. Beat the egg whites until stiff and gradually fold into the poi mixture. Put in a 1½ quart casserole. Bake uncovered for 30 minutes. Then brown at 425° F. for 5–10 minutes. Serve hot with turkey gravy.

Sesame Nut Cream

1 cup sesame milk
½ cup nut butter

6 pitted dates, chopped

Blend well and serve over breakfast fruit, or as a sweet dressing for salads.

Stuffing, Buckwheat

Sauté 5 minutes in 3 tablespoons fat:
1 onion
1 stalk celery

parsley

Add to 2 cups cooked buckwheat. If desired, 1 or 2 pimientos or mushrooms may be added. This is also good with ½ cup dried apricots added.

Stuffing, Rice

¼ cup chopped onion
2 cups cooked rice (natural brown, or wild)
Dash of salt

¼ teaspoon sage
¼ cup parsley and giblets (if desired)
½ cup chopped celery

Sauté onion and celery. Add to cooked rice. Moisten with chicken broth and season with salt and sage. Add parsley and giblets (if desired).

PANCAKES, WAFFLES, AND GRANOLA

Arrowroot Waffles
(wheat free, milk free)

1 cup arrowroot or tapioca or
    potato flour
3 eggs separated and beaten,
    whites very stiff
¼ cup water or less (add
    gradually)

2 tablespoons oil
2 tablespoons honey
¼ teaspoon sea salt

Add the flour to beaten yolks, then the oil, honey, and salt. Stir well and add water very gradually, the amount depending on the humidity. When smooth, fold in beaten whites and bake in thoroughly cleaned waffle iron. This is to remove any wheat flour residue. Permitted oil may be used to grease iron if necessary.

Artichoke Pancakes
(wheat free, milk free)

2 egg whites
2 egg yolks
1 cup arrowroot or tapioca starch

¼ cup artichoke starch
¼ cup water

Beat egg whites until stiff. Set aside. To egg yolks add arrowroot or tapioca starch, artichoke starch, and water. Beat well. Fold in egg whites. Drop by spoonfuls on hot pan. (Be sure to sift artichoke starch so it isn't lumpy.)

Pancakes
(grain free, egg free)

1 cup any starch
1 cup any seeds or nuts

Liquid as needed (water or milk
    substitute)

Blend the dry mixture at low speed adding liquid. Increase speed. Add only enough liquid to reach the right consistency.

Note: Because there is no leavening, the pancake will be flatter than usual. Therefore, the batter should be thicker than usual. As you experiment for the right consistency, remember that it is easier to add liquid than dry mixture. To grease the griddle, use the oil made from the seed or nut used. Example: sunflower oil with sunflower seeds, almond oil with almonds.

Granola

3 quarts oats	1 cup water
1 cup oat flour	⅓ cup almond oil
2 cups seeds	2 cups almonds

Preheat oven to 250° F. Mix oats, flour, seeds, and nuts. Add the combined oil and water. Stir well until everything is thoroughly coated. Use more water if needed or more oil if desired. The mixture should be a little moist. Spread evenly on cookie sheets. Bake for 30–40 minutes. Let cool on the sheets. Then store in ½ gallon or gallon jars.

Variations:

Sweeten with dried coconut.

Add 1 cup finely chopped dried apricots and/or 1 cup finely chopped dried peaches or cherries.

Buckwheat Pancakes 1
(wheat free, egg free, milk free)

1 cup buckwheat flour	1¼ cup water
1 teaspoon salt	

Stir well, then beat with an electric or hand beater until full of bubbles. Fry on well-greased griddle.

Buckwheat Pancakes 2
(wheat free, milk free)

1½ cup buckwheat flour	¾ teaspoon salt
2½ teaspoons baking powder	2 well-beaten eggs
2 tablespoons honey	5 tablespoons oil
¾ cup water	

Prepare as above.

Coconut Pancakes
(wheat free, milk free, egg free)

1¼ cups water	1 cup coconut meal
2 tablespoons vegetable oil	3 teaspoons baking powder
1 cup soy flour (or tolerated flour)	½ teaspoon salt

Put all ingredients in blender and blend until just mixed. Fry on well-greased griddle. If batter becomes too thick, add a small amount of water.

Carob Pancakes
(wheat free, milk free)

3 egg yolks
¼ cup water
3 tablespoons carob powder

1 cup arrowroot starch minus
    3 tablespoons
3 egg whites

Mix and fry without grease in electric fry pan (380° F.) Flip once (5–10 minutes).

New Hampshire Bannock
(wheat free, milk free, egg free)

1 cup whole white corn meal
2 tablespoons soft butter

½ teaspoon salt
boiling water

Preheat oven to 350° F. Combine corn meal and salt and pour over this enough boiling water to make a batter of the consistency of thick cream. Add butter. Spread thin in large well-greased pan. Bake about 45 minutes or until crispy brown. Delicious served with maple syrup or maple butter. Also good with soup.

Potato Pancakes
(wheat free, milk free)

4 large potatoes
1 egg

2 tablespoons potato meal

Peel and grate potatoes. Mix in meal and egg. On very low heat, oil pan; spoon mixture into pan. Brown and turn over. Serve alone or with apple or pear sauce.

Variation:

Place in oiled cake dish and bake in oven at very low heat until brown and cooked through.

Rice Waffles
(wheat free)

1½ cups rice flour
1 tablespoon baking powder
1 teaspoon salt
1½ cups milk

2 egg yolks, beaten
3 tablespoons melted fat or oil
2 egg whites, stiffly beaten

Mix dry ingredients well. Beat in milk, egg yolks, and fat. Fold in egg whites. Bake in hot waffle iron.

PIES

Most pie recipes are too complex for the person with many allergies. Therefore, we shall give one recipe and demonstrate how to make individual variations.

For the crust: use any nut, seed, or coconut meal, which can usually be purchased in health food stores. Meal can be made from any nut or seed by grinding nuts ½ cup at a time in a blender. For soft nuts (like cashews) use chop speed; for hard nuts, grind speed. (For ease of use, if you have an Osterizer, use an Oster jar instead of the blender container. If the Ball brand of Mason jar with the narrow mouth fits tightly on the blade, it can be substituted.)

The oil of the nuts causes those nearest the blade to lump together; separate these from the dry nuts in the center, using them for the bottom crust and saving the drier nuts for the top crust. The oily nuts may need an additional teaspoon or two of oil for the crust. (This depends on how oily the nut used and how long you kept it in the blender.)

Grease the pie plate lightly with oil and press the oily nuts or seeds or coconut ¼" thick, covering the bottom and the sides of the pan. (Eight heaping teaspoons give a generous crust for a small, deep-dish pie; about 2 cups are needed for a 9" pie.) Some people prefer a thinner crust. Add oil to part of the nut meal and then press the oily nuts, first with a spoon, then firmly with your thumbs. You must judge the amount of oil that will be needed and, if too much oil was used, add more nut meal. If you like it thicker, you can always add more nuts or seeds later.

On the following pages you will find a few recipes for crusts. If you can use grains, you'll have little difficulty finding a recipe for a grain crust. If you can tolerate none of these, you can try using a cookie recipe or a sponge cake recipe and use it as a crust, covering it with filling and serving as a shortcake. For the filling: 2 cups liquid; 2 tablespoons starch; fresh or frozen fruit (optional). The liquid may be any juice allowed (except citrus, for which you need a different recipe), any stewed fruit and/or frozen fruit which has been allowed to defrost and soak in its own juice. The starch may be arrowroot, tapioca, cornstarch, potato starch, rice flour, rye flour, artichoke flour. The first four are the best thickeners for fillings.

Pour the liquid over the starch, mixing thoroughly. Optional: Put on medium heat, stirring constantly, being very careful not to burn. As soon as it thickens, remove from heat. (A double boiler is the best way to heat filling.) Tapioca is one starch that thickens after it is removed from the heat. Remove and continue to stir. After the filling has cooled, place it over the bottom crust leaving room for fruit if you are using any. Cover the filling with the crushed dry nuts, seeds, coconut, or meringue. Cover with a Pyrex dish (to keep dry nuts from browning before bottom crust). Place in oven preheated to 400° F. for 20–40 minutes (or until the bottom crust is lightly browned).

Using rotation diet, here are three different pies:

	Monday	Tuesday	Wednesday
Crust	Almond	Filberts	Pecans
Fruit filling	Cherry juice and frozen oxhart cherries	Blueberry juice and frozen blueberries	Apple juice and partially cooked apples
Oil	Almond	Sesame	Safflower
Starch	Tapioca	Arrowroot starch	Cornstarch

Variations:

Use your own combinations.

Pie Crusts and Fillings

Almond-Wheat Pie Crust
(milk free, egg free)

1 cup flour
¼ cup ground almond meal
¼ cup oil (safflower, sunflower)

¼ cup maple syrup
½ teaspoon salt

Preheat oven to 375° F. Combine ingredients and press into pie dish to form crust. Bake until brown after filling has been added.

Barley Flour Pie Crust
(wheat free, milk free, egg free)

1½ cups whole barley flour
½ teaspoon salt

3–4 tablespoons water (ice cold)
4 tablespoons whole fat

Preheat oven to 400° F. Sift flour before measuring. Add salt and chop in fat with a pastry blender, gradually add water. Pie crust made from flour other than wheat is hard to handle so do not expect this to roll out as ordinary pie crust will. Roll it, then lift it into the pie pan and pat it into shape. Bake in quick oven 15 minutes.

Oatmeal Pie Crust
(wheat free)

1½ cups rolled oats   ¼ cup oil (rice bran or corn)
½ teaspoon salt   3 or 4 teaspoons water

Combine ingredients and press into crust in pie pan. Bake.

Oil Pie Crust

2 cups sifted flour   1½ teaspoons salt
½ cup oil (not olive)   ¼ cup cold water or milk

Preheat oven to 425° F. Do not mix. Add all ingredients at once to flour. Stir lightly until blended. Roll. It is easier to press the bottom into pie pan and to pat the top flat on a cutting board. Prick both top and bottom well with a fork. Fill. Bake 40 minutes. For shell or tart shells, bake at 475° F. for 10 minutes.

Variations:

Cheese: ⅔ cup grated cheddar to upper crust, otherwise as above.
   Nut: ½ cup ground nuts. Bake as above.
   Citrus: 2 tablespoons water and 2 tablespoons lemon juice instead of water (¼ cup). 1 teaspoon grated lemon or orange rind and ½ teaspoon honey added to dry ingredients.

Grape Pie Filling
(wheat free)

Boil white grapes in a little water to make juice. Put grapes through juicer, the seeds fly—watch out! For cleaner kitchen, use seedless grapes.

Boil:
½ cup grape juice   ½ cup maple syrup

Thicken with:
2 tablespoons arrowroot starch   2 tablespoons water

Nut Pastry
(wheat free, milk free)

½ cup ground nuts   ¾ teaspoon salt
½ cup water   1 teaspoon tapioca
1 cup oat flour

Preheat oven to 475° F. Mix ingredients. Press into pan. Bake 3–5 minutes. Fill crust with pie filling and continue baking.

Pecan Pie Filling
(wheat free, milk free)

Boil:
½ cup orange juice   ¼ cup pecan bits
¼ cup maple syrup

Thicken with:
2 tablespoons arrowroot starch   Dash of cinnamon
½ cup water   Dash of salt

Carob Pudding
(wheat free, egg free)

3¼ cups water, milk or milk   3 tablespoons butter (if allowed)
   substitute   Dash of salt
3 tablespoons potato starch   ¾ cup maple syrup
3 tablespoons carob

Mix to thicken. Stir while cooking.

SALADS

Salad Combinations

Try some of the following for salad combinations. If they don't fit into a rotation plan, invent combinations that do.

Tomatoes, sweet green pepper, and chopped peanuts.
Radishes, chopped peanuts, or hazelnuts.
Grated sweet potatoes, chopped sweet peppers, grated peanuts
Lettuce, grated coconut, macerated bananas
Pineapple and tomatoes
Cucumbers, onions, celery, and grated coconut
Tomatoes and cucumbers with vegetable dressing
Peas, cabbage, chopped nuts; mix with a teaspoon of honey
Pineapple and papaya
Apples, apple juice, nuts
Apples, apple juice, cabbage, nuts
Apples, celery and nuts
Chicken and avocado
Avocado and lemon juice

Apple-Celery Salad

2 tablespoons honey	1 cup chopped apple
2 tablespoons arrowroot starch	1 cup apple juice
1 cup chopped celery	

Heat apple juice and honey. Add arrowroot starch mixed with 2 tablespoons juice at room temperature. Cook and stir until thick and clear. Cool and add crisp celery and apple.

Cantaloupe Salad

Cut a cantaloupe in half. Stuff with a combination of fruits like sliced bananas, chopped pineapple, berries, and grated coconut.

Cabbage Salad 1

1 cup cabbage	1 cup carrot, grated
1 cup celery, diced	

Mix with olive oil or lemon juice.

Cabbage Salad 2

Mix equal parts of red and green cabbage with 1 small cucumber, diced; 1 cup chopped celery. Mix with mayonnaise.

Cole Slaw

Shred cabbage. Chop up grapefruit and toss with grapefruit juice.

Variation:

Use pineapple, apple, or orange.

Fruit Salad

Mix: strawberries, blueberries, raspberries, peaches, sliced bananas, grated fresh coconut, chopped walnuts.
Add honey if desired.

Guacamole

In a bowl, mash one avocado for each person. Add finely chopped onion, a clove of garlic, pressed. Mix thoroughly with lemon juice and olive oil.

Serve with crackers, or spread on lettuce, red cabbage, tomatoes, carrot sticks, or radishes.

Nut Loaf

1 cup carrots
½ cup chopped parsley
1 clove garlic

1 cup tomatoes, chopped
½ cup bell pepper, minced
2 tablespoons oil

Put through a food grinder. Now add ground peanuts or other nuts to form a loaf stiff enough to mold. Serve on platter and garnish with parsley and green onions. You may vary this recipe by adding sage, thyme, savory, or dill to the mixture.

Peach Salad

1 pound peaches
¼ pound pecans

1 firm ripe avocado

Slice peaches and mix with avocado. Mix with pecans. Serve with yogurt dressing.

Spinach Salad

½ cup spinach leaves, chopped
2 tablespoons chopped onion
1–2 teaspoons oil

½ cup beet leaves, chopped
2 teaspoons salad herbs
1 hard-cooked egg, chopped

Mix and serve.

Stringbean Salad

1 cup diced radishes or carrots
1 cup stringbeans, sliced thin

1 cup peanuts, almonds, or
   coconut

Mix and serve.

Waldorf Salad

Toss lightly together:
2 cups diced apples
1 cup chopped celery

½ cup chopped walnuts
½ cup seedless raisins

Mix with mayonnaise and serve on lettuce leaf.

SOUPS

Barley Water

4 tablespoons pearl barley
rind and juice of 2 lemons

1 quart water (4 cups)
honey to taste

Wash barley. Combine barley, water, and lemon rind and bring to a boil. Simmer for 2 hours. Strain and sweeten to taste. Add lemon juice to taste.

Chicken Gumbo Soup

One 4–4½ pound stewing chicken, cut up

2 cups water   ½ teaspoon salt

Cook until tender, about 2 hours. Remove chicken from bones and cube; skim fat from broth.

Combine and add:

4 cups thinly sliced okra	1 teaspoon honey
1 16-ounce can tomatoes, cut	2 teaspoons salt
½ cup chopped onion	⅛ teaspoon pepper

Cover and simmer ½ hour or until okra is tender. Serves 8.

Meat and Vegetable Soup

1 leg of lamb   4 or 5 quarts water

Remove most of the meat from leg of lamb (or other meat that has been slow roasted at 250° F.). Place bones in pan containing 4 or 5 quarts of cold water. Bring to boil and then allow to simmer (on low to medium heat) for about 12 hours. If you do not like your soup bland, cook it down to 2 quarts. (See Chapter 14 for instructions for removing fat and freezing.) When ready to eat, defrost, garnish with meat and vegetable. Salt to taste.

Variations:

1. Lamb with zucchini and fresh spearmint.
2. Ham with carrots, celery, and parsley (celery root if it is in season)
3. Moose with lima beans and tarragon
4. Buffalo with lentils or split peas

Instant Soup

Note: To make instant meat and vegetable soup, use cubes of meat gravy, three parts water to one part gravy (or the combination that suits your taste best). Garnish as above.

Split Pea or Lentil Soup

1–1½ cups lentils
2 or 3 carrots, diced
5 stalks chopped celery

½ pound mushrooms
1 quart water

Fill large saucepan with water. Add lentils (depending upon thickness desired) or dried peas and let soak overnight or for several hours. Cook slowly 1 hour; add carrots, celery, and mushrooms (unless allergic to yeast and other fungi). Salt well and cook for another hour, adding water when necessary.

Vegetable Meat Soup

2–4 cups diced, cooked meat
2 quarts (8 cups) seasoned stock
   or broth

1 or 2 quarts (4–8 cups) diced
   vegetables

This can be frozen after cooking, even with potatoes. With beef, use turnips if possible. Makes 8 or more servings.

SPROUTS

Seeds That May Be Sprouted. Alfalfa, beans, red clover, cress, fenugreek, lentils, mung bean, oats, parsley, dried peas, radish, rye, soy bean, sunflower, wheat, and almost any other seed that will grow.

Why Sprout Seeds? Seeds when sprouted are more easily digested. Patients allergic to some seeds can sometimes tolerate them when sprouted. The nutrient value sometimes increases with sprouting.

Methods for Growing Sprouts. Select good quality seeds—those not sprayed or treated with chemicals or preservatives.

A one or two quart wide-mouthed jar, is the simplest and most inexpensive to use. A piece of cotton gauze or a fine stainless steel screen should be held in place over the mouth of the jar by a rubber band or canning ring. For a 1-quart jar: Use one level tablespoon of alfalfa seed or 2 level tablespoons of mung beans (or larger seeds). Be sure to remove all broken or cracked seeds as they will only rot and spoil sprouts. Put in jar and cover with several inches of lukewarm water. Place net or cheesecloth over jar and secure with rubber band. Soak seeds overnight in a dark cupboard for about 5 hours. Drain and rinse well. Lay jar on its side in a fairly dark place for the first couple of days. However, be sure to rinse with lukewarm water 2 or 3 times daily. Flood jar and drain well each time. *Rinsing is the key to good sprouts.* As the seeds germinate they produce heat and waste which encourages the growth of bacteria. Thus they must be faithfully cooled and washed at least morning and evening to produce a tasty crop.

Rule: Keep them warm and moist all the time, but not wet. Cold delays growth. Too much heat encourages molding. When leaves begin to show (about the fourth day), allow light on jar. Place near window for more vitamin A and chlorophyll. When two green leaves have opened out fully, sprouts are at the height of their value and ready to use.

A quarter cup of mung beans will give you about 2 cups of bean sprouts.

When to Eat Sprouts. Alfalfa sprouts taste best when 1" to 2" long. Mung beans are best when 1½" to 3" long. Wheat sprouts are most delicious when the sprout is the length of the seed. Lentil sprouts are edible within 36 hours; should be used when about 1" long. Sunflower seed sprouts are best when no longer than the seed. Pea and soybean sprouts are good short or long. When sprouts have developed to the desired stage, put in a glass jar in refrigerator. They will keep for several days if properly covered. Alfalfa sprouts take about 5 days or so to develop, mung beans about 4 or 5 days. Wheat and lentil sprouts are ready in about 2 days.

Alfalfa Sprouts. These should never be cooked. Snack on them as is. Mix a handful with favorite spread, tahini, sesame butter, mayonnaise. Add to salads, cottage cheese, soup, or stew just before serving. Excellent for sandwiches in place of lettuce and a lot cheaper.

Alfalfa Sprout Toss

2 cups finely cut celery	1 cup raisins
1 cup sprouted alfalfa	2 carrots, grated

Mix thoroughly and when ready to serve, make a "dent" in top of salad to fill with generous amounts of thick yogurt or sour cream.

Alfalfa Sprouts Milk

2 cups fruit juice	2 tablespoons nuts
1 cup alfalfa sprouts	honey to taste

Place ingredients in blender and liquefy.

Avocado Alfalfa

1 cubed avocado	alfalfa sprouts
3 cups vegetables (cut in chunks)	

Toss avocado and vegetables. Add alfalfa sprouts. No dressing is needed. Avocado replaces dressing.

Variations:

Take 1 ripe tomato and cut from top to bottom but not through bottom. Set and spread slightly on mound of alfalfa sprouts. Fill center of tomato with scoop of mashed avocado to which has been added a few drops of lemon juice and salt.

Substitute green pepper.

Lentil Sprouts

Lentil sprouts are good when added to soups just before serving. May be prepared plain, with herbs, tomato sauce, diced onions, or any seasoning desired.

Mung Bean Sprouts

One of the highest vegetable protein foods. Eaten raw, they taste like fresh pod peas. Add to omelets, soups.

Seed Butter

1 cup sesame or sunflower seeds   1 tablespoon oil
vegetable seasoning

Grind or blend repeatedly until fine and smooth. Store in refrigerator.

Wheat Balls

1 cup sprouted wheat   salt to taste
1 cup nuts   2 cups dry fruit or fresh fruits

Grind all ingredients in blender, add the salt and mix. Make into 1″ balls and roll in fresh shredded coconut. Use as a dessert.

VEGETABLES

Almond Asparagus

Preheat oven to 350° F. Alternate layers of cooked asparagus in oiled casserole with grated cheese and toasted blanched almonds. Bake 20 minutes.

Eggplant Parmigiana

1 eggplant (about 2 pounds)   oregano to taste (optional)
¼ cup grated cheese   ¾ cup oil and butter mixed
½ pound brick cheese   1½ cups tomato sauce

Preheat oven to 400° F. Peel eggplant and cut into ¼" slices. Brush both sides with oil and butter. Broil. Drain on towel if desired. Put layer of eggplant slices in shallow baking dish. Cover with tomato sauce, a little grated cheese, and a few slices of brick cheese. Repeat layers until all ingredients are used ending with sliced cheese. Bake uncovered 15 minutes, or until mixture is thoroughly heated. Be careful not to over-bake as it toughens the cheese.

Jerusalem Artichokes

Prepare by scrubbing and then scraping or peeling thinly. Put at once in cold water to cover, with 1 tablespoon vinegar or lemon juice to each quart to keep good color. Leave in the water ½ hour. (This step may be omitted if they are sliced ⅓"–¼" thick and steamed. Steaming time about 5–6 minutes.) Cook by putting into boiling salted water to cover and simmer until tender, about 20–30 minutes. Overcooking makes them soggy.

Boil in jackets and peel them afterwards.

Roast them.

Broil them like potato crisps.

To serve, make a sauce, using some of the cooking water. Or serve au gratin. Or use for soup or stew. Or serve cold in salad. Or simply serve lightly salted, with or without butter.

Legumes

1½ cups of dried beans will serve 6. Split peas, lentils, pinto beans, and blackeyed peas can be cooked without soaking. Other dried legumes should be soaked. Some double in size, lentils more than double, soybeans increase three times their original size.

To retain nutritive value and develop full natural flavor, simmer legumes in the water in which they were soaked.

Soybeans are an excellent substitute for meat since ½ cup provides 10 units of protein and only 105 calories. The protein in other legumes is incomplete and must be supplemented with eggs, cheese, milk, meat, grains or sesame seeds.

Okra, Boiled

Drop into boiling water. With lid on cook 4–5 minutes. Salt and butter or season with vinegar and salt.

Okra, Broiled

Southern style. Cut okra into small pieces (about ¼″ thick). Roll in beaten egg, then roll in starch (arrowroot, tapioca) or flour. Brush with oil and broil at a low heat.

Okra, Steamed

Okra is good used in soup or cooked with tomatoes. Steam until tender. Season with 2 tablespoons oil, salt, and 1 teaspoon of the herb of your choice.

Peppers, Stuffed

1 quart tomato juice   2 green peppers
1 pound chopped meat   dash of salt

Preheat oven to 350° F. Roll meat into balls 1″ in diameter and place in a covered saucepan filled with tomato juice. Let simmer at very low heat for hours (until juice has turned to sauce). Salt to taste. Core green peppers and blanch by parboiling for 2 minutes. Fill the green peppers with the thickened sauce and meat and bake in covered dish 15 minutes.

Pickles, Canned Fresh

Fill sterilized jars with small cucumber pickles, 2 cloves of garlic (optional), 1 piece fresh dill, 1 teaspoon salt, and ½ teaspoon celery seed (optional).

Boil 2 parts water to 1 part apple cider vinegar. (Pour over pickles and cap; tighten lid.) Put in cold bath until it comes to a boil, when small bubbles appear (approximately 20 minutes). Take out and check for dark green spots. If there are any, put back for a few more minutes. Take out, let stand and tighten lids.

Variation:

Add ½ teaspoon mustard seed.

Plantain, Broiled

1 plantain   1 cup oil

Cut plantain in rounds. Brush with oil and broil at low heat. Either green or ripe plantain may be used. Green plantain makes a good biscuit substitute. Ripe plantain is sweet. It is good served with the meal or as a dessert.

Potato Puffs
(wheat free)

½ cup whole potato flour
⅛ teaspoon salt
2 teaspoons baking powder

1½ teaspoons melted whole fat or
   1 teaspoon oil
1 egg
½ cup milk

Preheat oven to 375° F. Sift flour before measuring. Mix dry ingredients. Add fat or oil. Beat egg, add milk and combine with dry ingredients. Bake in muffin pans 25 minutes.

Spinach

Don't *always* cook the spinach. Tear up the raw leaves and season with your favorite herbal vinegar salad dressing. Discard watery stems.

Squash, Butternut, Oatmeal

Boil and puree equal amounts of butternut squash and oatmeal. May add nutmeg for flavor. Makes a custard.

Squash, Winter

Cut hard-shelled squash into serving pieces; place in steamer or improvised steamer flesh side down (skin up) and steam until tender. Reverse on cookie sheet, spread with dark molasses and/or butter, oil, and meat (sausage or ground beef seasoned with herbs, partially cooked bacon). Brown lightly under broiler and serve.

Zucchini, Stuffed

6″–8″ zucchini
2 tablespoons cheese
1 quart water

1 cup creamed, chopped (fresh or
   frozen) spinach, broccoli,
   chard (or a combination of
   these)

Preheat oven to 350° F. Cook zucchini in boiling water until tender (7–8 minutes). Drain. Cut lengthwise, scoop out centers. Drain again. Sprinkle shell with salt and stuff with the centers of the zucchini mixed with any of above vegetables or combination of these vegetables. Place stuffed zucchini in a greased shallow baking pan or oven-to-table dish. Sprinkle each portion with cheese. Before serving, reheat in the oven about 20 minutes.

Notes

Chapter 1

1. Lawrence Dickey, ed., *Clinical Ecology* (Springfield, Ill.: Charles C Thomas, 1970).
2. Theron G. Randolph, *Human Ecology and Susceptibility to the Chemical Environment* (Springfield, Ill.: Charles C Thomas, 1962).

Chapter 2

1. Doris J. Rapp, *Allergies and the Hyperactive Child* (New York: Sovereign, 1979).

Chapter 3

1. Theron G. Randolph, *Human Ecology and Susceptibility to the Chemical Environment*. This is described in detail as "Decrease in Adaptation."
2. This example was cited to us by Dr. Marshall Mandell.
3. Dr. Joseph Morgan of Coos Bay, Oregon is a past president of the Society for Clinical Ecology.

Chapter 5

1. Dr. David Hawkins of Manhasset, New York, and Dr. Carl C. Pfeiffer of Princeton, New Jersey, are members of the editorial board for the Journal of Orthomolecular Psychiatry, the official journal of the Academy of Orthomolecular Psychiatry. Publication Office, 2231 Broad Street, Regina, Saskatchewan, Canada S4P 1Y7.
2. We are grateful to Dr. Bell, who, at the time it was being presented for publication, gave permission to quote from her paper, "Food and Chemical Factors in Sleep Disorders."
3. This case was reported by Dr. Marshall Mandell at the meeting of the International Academy of Preventive Medicine, Kansas City, Mo., October 12, 1973.

Chapter 7

1. Hans Selye, *The Stress of Life* (New York: McGraw-Hill, 1956).
2. We wish to express our gratitude to Dr. James C. Cox, a pastoral counselor, who, recognizing our need for body therapy, exercise, and relaxation methods, personally trained us in the physical therapies he practiced and who introduced us to professionals for training in other physical modalities.

Chapter 9

1. We are grateful to Jane Roller (M.Sc. in Botany from Ohio State University) who compiled these lists using the following references: L. H. Bailey, *The Standard Cyclopedia of Horticulture.* (New York: The Macmillan Company, 1941); H. H. Collins Jr., *Complete Guide to American Wildlife* (New York: Harper and Brothers, 1959); T. H. Everett, ed., *New Illustrated Encyclopedia of Gardening* (New York: Greystone Press, 1960); R. H. Manville, *Plants Used as Food by Man* and *Animals Commonly Eaten by Man.* Mimeo, Eugene W. Higgins, M.D., Washington, D.C., 1968; H. J. Rinkel, T. G. Randolph, and M. Zeller, *Food Allergy* (Springfield, Ill.: Charles C. Thomas, 1951).

Chapter 11

1. Aron Streit, Inc., 148–154 Rivington St., New York, N.Y. 10002.
2. Dr. Marshall Mandell cautions the public to question their pharmacists about side effects of their medication. You have a right to see the literature published by the manufacturer. We are grateful to Dr. Mandell who has written and lectured extensively on the relationship between molds and cerebral allergies.

Chapter 12

1. Dr. Lawrence Dickey of Fort Collins, Colorado, is a past president of the Society for Clinical Ecology, the Program Director for the Seminars on Clinical Ecology and the editor of the textbook *Clinical Ecology.* We wish to thank Dr. Dickey who graciously took the time to teach us the concept of the rotary diversified diet as he practices it.
2. Catherine Elwood, *Feel Like a Million* (New York: Pocket Books, 1970).
3. *Composition of Foods: Raw, Processed, and Prepared.* Agriculture Handbook, no. 8 (Washington, D.C.: U.S. Department of Agriculture, 1963).

Chapter 13

1. Alsop Corwin, A.B., Ph.D., D.Sc.: Professor of Chemistry, Emeritus, The Johns Hopkins University, Baltimore, Maryland.
2. Walnut Acres: Penns Creek, Pennsylvania 17862.
3. Cellophane bags: Nuvita Food Co., 7524 S. W. Macadam Ave., Portland, Oregon.
4. Dine-out Cartons: P.O. Box 702, Neenah, Wisconsin 54951.

Chapter 18

1. When this problem was discovered, it was Francis Silver who found the solution and shared it with us.
2. International Baseboard Heat, Intertherm Hot Water Division. Intertherm, Inc., 3800 Park Ave., St. Louis, Missouri 63110; phone (314) 771–2419.

3. Kennedy Natural Food Store, 1051 West Broad St., Falls Church, Virginia 22046, phone (703) 533-8484. They issue a catalog and ship by United Parcel Service. We are very grateful to the Kennedys who also helped us locate special items such as fish nail files for those sensitive to emery boards and the Loofa, a natural plant body brush, real sponges, and other nontoxic products so difficult to find.

Chapter 19

1. Dr. Del Stigler, Secretary of the Society for Clinical Ecology, 2005 Franklin, Suite 490, Denver, Colorado 80205.
2. See note 3, Chap. 13.
3. When not available locally, write for catalog: Garden Kitchens, 270 West Merrick Road, Valley Stream, N.Y. 11582.
4. See note 3, Chap. 13.
5. Rokeach coconut oil soap. To find local distributor write: Rokeach and Sons, Farmingdale, New Jersey 07727.

Chapter 23

1. See note 2, Chap. 18.
2. Puro Filter Corporation. Main office: 20–01 51 Ave., Long Island City, N.Y. 11101.

Chapter 24

1. Oakite. For distributor nearest you, write: Oakite, 50 Valley Road, Berkley Heights, New Jersey 07922.

Chapter 26

1. Ecologists Cotton Co-op, 2986 Talisman Drive, Dallas, Texas 75229.

Chapter 27

1. We are indebted to Francis Silver, who furnished these cases and taught us these practices.

Chapter 29

1. A particular note of gratitude is due to Dr. Joseph Morgan, whose efforts in the area of travel proved very helpful.
2. Write: Air Conditioning Engineers, P.O. Box 616, Decatur, Ill. 62525.
3. Eddie Bauer, P.O. Box 3700, Seattle, Washington 98124; or Norm Thompson, 1805 N.W. Thurman, Portland, Oregon 97209.
4. To locate address of local distributor of Zer-O-Ice, write to R.M. Hollings-

head Corp., Camden, New Jersey 08102. Metal canned ice is also available from Classic Chemical, 1101 Avenue G., Arlington, Texas 76011.

Chapter 30

1. Dr. Michael Schachter of Nyack, New York is an orthomolecular psychiatrist who has incorporated clinical ecology into his practice.

Bibliography and Source Materials

The following publications and sources are suggested as aids in solving the daily problems encountered in the altered life style of the person with food and/or chemical allergies. They can also be a source of medical information for skeptical husbands, wives, relatives, friends, and even doctors.

Composition of Foods: Raw, Processed, and Prepared. Agriculture Handbook, no. 8, U.S. Department of Agriculture, 1963. (Available from Superintendent of Documents, U.S. Government Printing Office, Washington, D.C. 20402.) Comprehensive tables of the nutrient contents of various foods.

Crook, William G. *Can Your Child Read? Is He Hyperactive?* Jackson, Tenn.: Pedicenter Press, 1975.

Dickey, Lawrence, ed. *Clinical Ecology.* Springfield, Ill.: Charles C. Thomas, 1970.
A comprehensive study for the professional.

Forman, Jonathan, *Soil, Food and Health.* Atlanta, Texas, P.O. Box 210, 1961.

Goldstein, Jerome, and Goldman, M.C., eds. *Guide to Organic Food Shopping and Organic Living.* Emmaus, Pa.: Rodale Press, Inc., 1970.
Directory of organic food sources listed by state.

Hall, Ross Hume, *Food for Naught, the Decline in Nutrition.* New York: Harper and Row, 1974.

Hunter, Beatrice Trum, *Consumer Beware.* New York: Simon & Schuster, 1971.
———, *Gardening Without Poisons.* Boston: Houghton-Mifflin Company, 2nd ed., 1971.
———, *Mirage of Safety: Food Additives and Federal Policy.* New York: Charles Scribner's Sons, 1976.
———, *The Great Nutrition Robbery.* New York: Charles Scribner's Sons, 1978.

Jensen, Bernard, D.C., *Nuts for You.* Escondido, Calif.: Hidden Valley Health Ranch, Route 6, Box 822.
———, *Seeds and Sprouts for Life.* Escondido, Calif.: Hidden Valley Health Ranch, Route 6, Box 822.

Kailin, Eloise W., and Brooks, Clifton R., "Systemic Toxic Reactions to Soft Plastic Food Containers: A Double-blind Study." Medical Annals of the District of Columbia, vol. 32, no. 1, January 1963.

MacKarness, Richard, *Eating Dangerously: The Hazards of Hidden Allergies*. New York and London: Harcourt Brace Jovanovich, 1976.

Miller, Joseph, *Something About Food Allergy: The Provocative Testing and Injection Therapy*. Springfield, Ill.: Charles C. Thomas, 1972.

Organic Gardening. Emmaus, Pa.: Rodale Press, Inc.

Randolph, Theron G., *Human Ecology and Susceptibility to the Chemical Environment*. Springfield, Ill.: Charles C. Thomas, 1962. Comprehensive discussion of sources of chemical contamination of air (indoor and outdoor), ingestants (food and drink), personal contacts (such as cosmetics), and treatment.

Rapp, Doris J., *Allergies and the Hyperactive Child*. New York: Sovereign, 1979.

Rinkel, H. J.; Randolph, T. G.; and Zeller, M., *Food Allergy*. 1951. Reprinted by New England Foundation of Allergic and Environmental Diseases, 3 Brush St., Norwalk, Conn. 06850.

Roberts, Rex, *Your Engineered House*. New York: M. Evans Company, 1964.

Rodale Press, *The Basic Book of Organically Grown Foods*. New York: New American Library, 1973.

ASSOCIATIONS AND THEIR PUBLICATIONS
(All are concerned with food allergies and/or chemical intolerances.)

1. *The Human Ecology Action League* (HEAL)
   505 N. Lakeshore Dr.
   Suite 6506
   Chicago, Ill. 60611

   An organization that represents the aims and programs of patients, physicians and others interested in environmental health.

   Publication:
   Human Ecologist. Published 6 times a year

2. *Human Ecology Study Group*
   Metropolitan Chicago Area Chapter of HEAL
   5460 N. Marmora
   Chicago, Ill. 60630

   A self-help organization for people with food allergies and/or chemical intolerances.

Publications:
  Very Basically Yours Cookbook, rev. Recipes, food substitutions, lists of foods containing milk, wheat, egg, corn, yeast, infant feeding, organic food brands, and food families. 100 pp.
  Housing Guide-1968—Advice on construction, painting, paneling, and furnishings. 5 pp.
  The Realities of Food Addiction.
  "Description and Recognition"
  "Treatment and Prophylaxis"
  Two pamphlets by Theron G. Randolph, M.D.
  Corn-Free List. List of common corn contacts.

3. *Society for Clinical Ecology*
   Del Stigler, M.D., Secretary
   2005 Franklin, Suite 490
   Denver, Colorado 80205

   A group of physicians, scientists and other professionals who are concerned about the effect of the total environment, particularly volatile hydrocarbons from solvents, plastics, insecticides, and similar agents, on sensitive people.
   Meetings: annual advanced seminars, basic seminars.
   Dues: $50 per year

Publications: The Archives of the Society, available to members.

4. *Allergy Foundation of Lancaster County*
   Box 1424, Lancaster, Pa., 17604

   A nonprofit tax-free organization devoted to a better scientific understanding and treatment of allergic diseases.

   Publications: by Stephen D. Lockey, M.D.:
     Elimination List for Individuals Clinically Sensitive to Aspirin
     Elimination List for Individuals Clinically Sensitive to Phenolphthalein
     Write for information about additional publications.

5. *New England Foundation for Allergic and Environmental Diseases*
   3 Brush Street, Norwalk, Connecticut 06850

   A nonprofit, tax-free organization devoted to research, dissemination of information and treatment of allergic and environmental diseases.

Publications:
  "Air Pollution: Cerebral Manifestation of Hypersensitivity to the Chemical Environment," by Marshall Mandell, M.D. Montreal, Quebec, Canada, 1967.
  "Allergic-Ecologic-Metabolic Factors in Physical and Mental Illness," reprinted from *New Dimensions of Preventive Medicine,* 1974.
  "Allergies Alleged to be Cause of Psychosis," reprinted from *Medical World,* 1970.
  Write for information about additional publications.

6. *The Human Ecology Research Foundation*
   720 N. Michigan Avenue, Chicago, Ill. 60611

   Supports medical research, application, and publication in the field of human ecology; source for reprints of Dr. Theron G. Randolph's numerous articles describing the relationships between chronic physical and mental illnesses, and food, drugs, and chemicals in the environment.

   Publications:
   Annual Report to Members
   Bibliography in *Bulletin* of the Human Ecology Research Foundation, #181, July 1967, 39 pp., Theron G. Randolph, M.D., ed.
   Extensive bibliography for the areas of environmental causes, bodily responses (obesity, alcoholism, localized allergies, constitutional responses, ecologic mental illness), cellular level investigations and theories, general adaptation, and ecology.
   The following reprinted articles from the above *Bibliography* might prove helpful:
   #166 Clinical Manifestations of Individual Susceptibility to Insecticides and Related Materials, 1965.
   #131 Ecologic Mental Illness—Levels of Central Nervous System Reactions, 1961.
   #160 Ecologic Orientation in Medicine: Comprehensive Environmental Control in Diagnosis and Therapy, 1965.
   #161 Food Addiction, Obesity, and Alcoholism, 1964.
   Air Pollution in the Schools and Its Effects on our Children, Kathleen A. Blume, 1968, 67 pp.
   Lists major causes and gives recommendations.

7. Human Ecology Research Foundation of the Southwest
   8345 Walnut Hill Lane, Suite 240, Dallas, Texas 75231

   Publications:
   Environmentally Triggered Phlebitis
   Environmentally Triggered Vasculitis
   Environmentally Triggered Heart Diseases
   Write for information about additional publications.

Index